Practical Skills Manual
for Evaluation
of Athletic Injuries

Practical Skills Manual for Evaluation of Athletic Injuries

William R. Holcomb, PhD, ATC, CSCS*D

Athletic Training Program Director
Department of Kinesiology
University of Nevada, Las Vegas

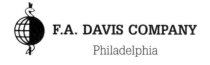

F.A. DAVIS COMPANY
Philadelphia

F. A. Davis Company
1915 Arch Street
Philadelphia, PA 19103
www.fadavis.com

Acquisitions Editor: Christa Fratantoro
Developmental Editor: Maryann Foley
Production Editor: Jack Brandt
Designer: Rita Naughton
Cover Designer: Louis Forgione

As new scientific information becomes available through basic and clinical research, recommended treatments and drug therapies undergo changes. The author(s) and publisher have done everything possible to make this book accurate, up to date, and in accord with accepted standards at the time of publication. The authors, editors, and publisher are not responsible for errors or omissions or for consequences from application of the book, and make no warranty, expressed or implied, in regard to the contents of the book. Any practice described in this book should be applied by the reader in accordance with professional standards of care used in regard to the unique circumstances that may apply in each situation. The reader is advised always to check product information (package inserts) for changes and new information regarding dose and contraindications before administering any drug. Caution is especially urged when using new or infrequently ordered drugs.

Library of Congress Cataloging in Publication Data

Holcomb, William.
    Practical skills manual for evaluation of athletic injuries / William Holcomb.
        p. cm.
    ISBN 0-8036-0784-9
    1. Sports injuries—Handbooks, manuals, etc. I. Title.

RD97 .H65 2002
617.1′027—dc21

                                                                2001054793

To my wonderful family, Our Father, Mom, Dad, Gdad, U. Bill, Libba, Phil, Dylan, Gaines, Julie, Ian, the Sanders, and great friends: Tim, Craig, Rich, Mike, Chris, Bill, Dick, Mark, Jutta, and Heather. Thanks for all your support.

Acknowledgments

I would like to take this opportunity to thank all of the wonderful staff at F.A. Davis who made the publication of this book possible. First, I would like to thank Jean-Francois Vilain, who served as the Publisher until his retirement in 2000. I would like to thank my Developmental Editors, Maryann Foley and Sharon Lee, for their patience in working with an inexperienced author. I would also like to thank Christa Fratantoro, Acquisitions Editor, for providing direction in the later stages of development.

I relied heavily on the work of other authors who have published textbooks with F.A. Davis. I would like to thank each of these authors for the figures and other work that I borrowed.

I would like to thank the following individuals for their careful review of this book:

Scott T. Doberstein, MS, LATC, CSCS, Head Athletic Trainer/Lecturer, Department of Exercise and Sports Science, University of Wisconsin–La Crosse, La Crosse, Wisconsin

Sheri Lee Martin, MPT, OCS, ATC, Orthopedic Clinical Specialist, Department of Athletic Training, Northeastern University, Boston, Massachusetts

Charles M. Rozanski, Jr., MEd, ATC, Director of Sports Medicine, North Carolina State University, Raleigh, North Carolina

Contents

Introduction

Assessment of athletic injuries is one of the major responsibilities of the athletic trainer. The primary purpose of this assessment is to determine the type and severity of injury so that the proper treatment or disposition can be provided. However, if done poorly, the consequences can be great.

Several plans have been developed to assist the athletic trainer in performing a thorough assessment to ensure proper recognition of athletic injuries. One popular plan is the *History, Observation, Palpation, Special tests* (HOPS) format. During the history portion of the assessment, the athletic trainer asks questions to identify the mechanism of injury and find out what the patient is experiencing. In the observation section, the athletic trainer inspects the part visually and then explores with palpation. Special tests are then used on the injured area to determine the type and severity of injury.

Another assessment strategy is the *Subjective, Objective, Assessment, Plan* (SOAP) format. Using this format, the athletic trainer obtains information from the injured patient by asking questions (subjective) and then by making observations free of input from the patient (objective). Based on this information, the athletic trainer then identifies the problem (assessment) and develops strategies to manage the injury at hand (plan).

These assessment formats have been used effectively by athletic trainers and other allied health professionals in recognizing athletic injuries. However, for the purpose of athletic training education, these strategies present some difficulty for students because many assessment techniques are combined under a single area. For example, HOPS uses special tests as the final step in the assessment. This section would include tests for fracture, range of motion (ROM), joint stability, and neurologic function. Therefore, to facilitate skill development in assessing athletic injuries, this practical skills manual is based on an expanded assessment strategy in which the areas of the assessment have been narrowed as follows:

1. History
2. Inspection
3. Palpation
4. ROM tests—active range of motion (AROM), passive range of motion (PROM), and resisted range of motion (RROM)
5. Joint stability tests
6. Special tests
7. Neurologic tests

The purpose of this manual is to provide students with guided activities to improve practical skills used in the assessment. It is recommended that students read their textbook and attend classroom lectures before completing the laboratory activities. These activities will help students develop skills that can be used to assess actual injuries during their supervised clinical experiences. An answer key is provided for selected activities that require students to provide written information before performing the given activities.

Practical Questions

The final activity in each chapter, Practical Questions, includes examination and performance questions that can be used to test practical assessment skills. After students complete the laboratory activities, a laboratory partner, clinical instructor, or classroom instructor can administer the practical questions. Performance evaluation sheets are provided to address the important components of the skill that is being assessed. Some items require only a simple check if the student gives an appropriate response, such as naming the test, giving positive signs, or using correct positioning. However, other components, such as the actual performance of a test or description of a test, can be graded, for example, on a numerical scale from 1 to 10, depending on the quality of the answer. A grade of 7 or higher would be considered a passing score.

Chapter 1

Developing General Assessment Skills

Errors in Terminology Usage
Medical vs. Layperson Terminology
Imaging Techniques

ANSWER KEY

Activity 7

ACTIVITY 1   Terms of Direction to Locate Anatomical Landmarks

Introduction

The ability to describe the location of an injury using anatomical terms is a basic assessment skill. Review the list of anatomical terms before completing the following exercise.

- **Medial**   Toward the midline of the body.
- **Lateral**   Away from the midline of the body.
- **Anterior/ventral**   Front.
- **Posterior/dorsal**   Back.
- **Superior/cephalad**   Toward the head.
- **Inferior/caudal**   Away from the head.
- **Proximal**   Nearer to the trunk.
- **Distal**   Farther from the trunk.
- **Superficial**   Near the surface.
- **Deep**   Away from the surface.
- **Supra**   Above.
- **Infra**   Below.

Instructions ➤   Locate and palpate each of the following surface anatomical landmarks illustrated on Figure 1–1. Using anatomical terminology, write a brief description of the location of each landmark. You may use other prominent structures in your description. There are several correct descriptions for each. A good description is one that directs a person to the named structure. The first description is done for you.

Base of fifth metatarsal	**Proximal** end of **lateral**most metatarsal
Olecranon process	_____
Medial malleolus	_____
Metacarpals	_____
Head of fibula	_____
Gastrocnemius	_____
Patella	_____
Vastus medialis	_____
Tibial tuberosity	_____
Rectus femoris	_____
Greater trochanter	_____
Ischial tuberosity	_____

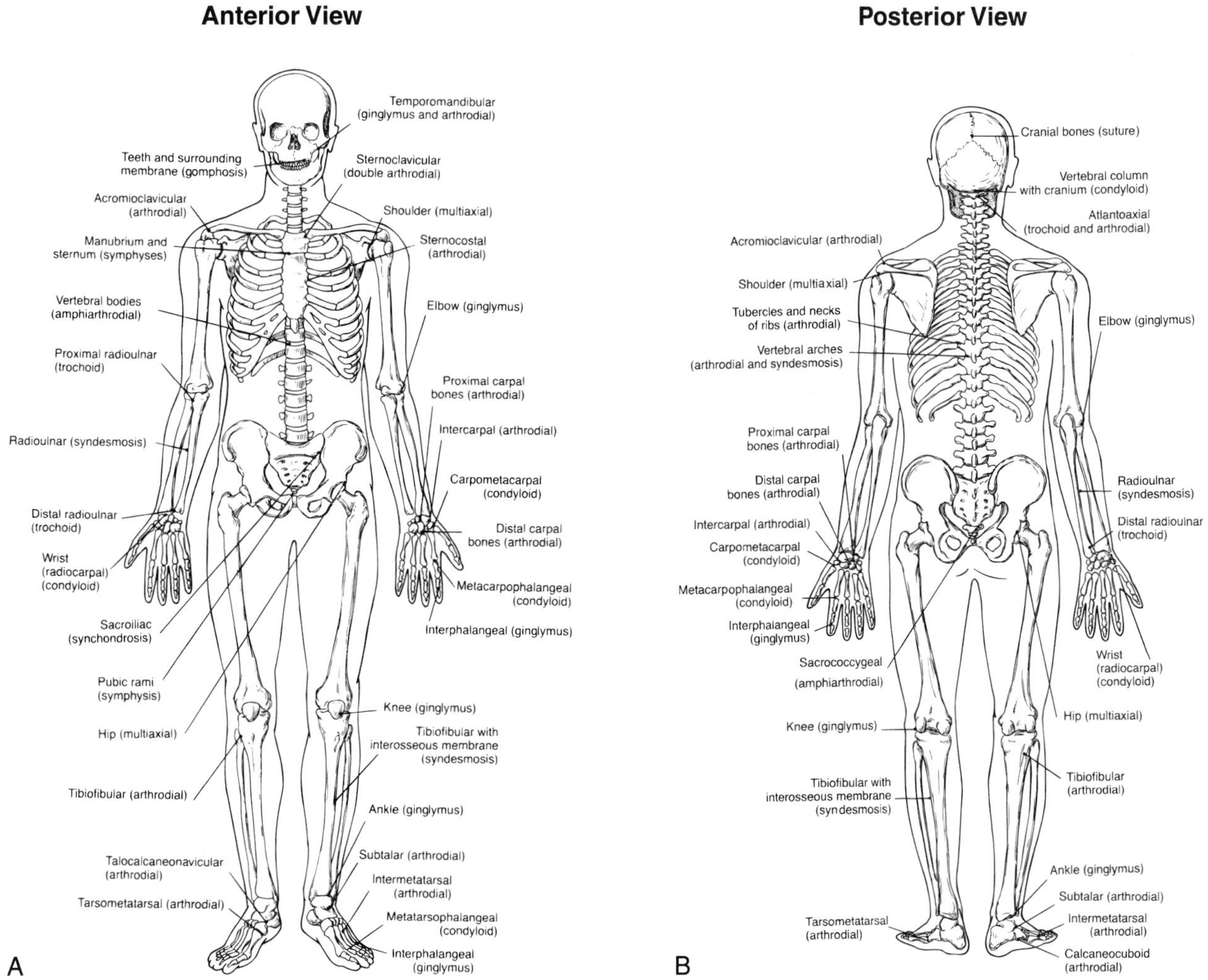

Anterior View

Posterior View

Figure 1–1 Anterior *(A)* and posterior *(B)* views of the body. (From Rothstein, JM, et al: The Rehabilitation Specialist's Handbook, ed 2. FA Davis, Philadelphia, 1998, pp 106–107, with permission.)

Anterior superior iliac spine _____

Gluteus maximus _____

Sternum _____

Erector spinae _____

Acromion process _____

Spine of scapula _____

Coracoid process _____

Anatomical snuffbox _____

Occipital protuberance _____

Maxilla _____

Mandible _____

Tarsal navicular _____

Thenar eminence _____

Hypothenar eminence _____

Lateral epicondyle _____

Hamate _____

ACTIVITY 2   The History Portion of an Assessment

Introduction

The history is one of the most difficult parts of the assessment to master. The purpose of the history is to gather information about the injury to guide the examiner in the remainder of the assessment. It is difficult to teach the technique of history taking because there is not a simple list of questions that are appropriate for all injuries. Therefore activities are included to help the student develop the skills needed to gather information about the history of an injury. A thorough, yet concise, history will help narrow the focus of the evaluation, thereby leading the clinician to limit the possible injuries to a specific few.

The history should include questions that will provide information about the following:

- Mechanism of injury
- Onset of injury
- Location of injury
- Description of pain
- Description of other symptoms
- What makes symptoms worse, what relieves symptoms
- Previous history of injury
- Previous treatment
- Functional ability
- Change in equipment
- Change in training

In addition to knowing the important questions to ask, knowing what the response indicates and knowing how to use this information in the remainder of the assessment are equally important. To improve your ability to ask appropriate questions and interpret responses, you will be asked to perform activities involving questions designed to elicit the appropriate response.

In this exercise you will serve as the evaluator and your partner will act as the injured patient. Your partner chooses an acute or chronic injury for the body part being studied. Your assignment is to ask specific questions that will provide the information described earlier in this section. Your partner's assignment is to give the answer that would be expected from a patient experiencing this injury. Write your questions and your partner's answers in the spaces provided so that you can analyze and discuss the quality of your effort with your partner and other students.

To further illustrate, an example of history taking for a grade 2 inversion ankle sprain follows:

Question: What happened?
Response: When I planted my foot, I turned my ankle (inverted my ankle).

Question: Did you hear any sounds when you were injured?
Response: No.

Question: Where does it hurt? Please point to the area of greatest pain with one finger.
Response: The patient points just anterior or inferior to the lateral malleolus.

Question: Describe the sensation at the time of injury and what you are experiencing now.
Response: I felt a sharp pain when I turned my ankle, and now I feel a dull ache.

Question: Do you feel a sensation other than pain?
Response: It feels very tight.

Question: What makes your ankle feel better, and what makes it feel worse?
Response: It hurts to stand or turn my foot in. It feels better to elevate my foot.

Question: Have you hurt your ankle before?
Response: I did the same thing before, but it didn't hurt this bad.

Question: What did you do for the earlier injury?
Response: My athletic trainer applied ice and a wrap and taped me for a couple of games.

Instructions ➤ Have your partner select a common acute injury from the body part that you are studying. Ask a series of questions in an attempt to narrow the injury possibilities and guide the assessment. Your partner should provide the answers that would be likely from a patient with this injury. Record both the questions and responses and discuss your conclusions with your partner and instructor. Repeat this process for a chronic injury, soft tissue injury, bony injury, and neurovascular pathology.

Acute Injury

Question: _____

Response: _____

Question: _____

Response: _____

Question: _____

Response: _____

Question: _____

Response: _____

Question: _____

Response: _____

Question: _____

Response: _____

Question: _____

Response: _____

Question: _____

Response: _____

Question: _____

Response: _____

Question: _____

Response: _____

Question: _____

Response: _____

Chronic Injury

Question: _____

Response: _____

Question: _____

Response: _____

Question: _____

Response: _____

Question: _____

Response: _____

Question: _____

Response: _____

Question: _____

Response: _____

Question: _____

Response: _____

Question: _____

Response: _____

Question: _____

Response: _____

Question: _____

Response: _____

Question: _____

Response: _____

Soft Tissue Injury

Question: _____

Response: _____

Question: _____

Response: _____

Question: _____

Response: _____

Question: _____

Response: _____

Question: _____

Response: _____

Question: _____

Response: _____

Question: _____

Response: _____

Question: _____

Response: _____

Question: _____

Response: _____

Question: _____

Response: _____

Question: _____

Response: _____

Bony Injury

Question: _____

Response: _____

Question: _____

Response: _____

Question: _____

Response: _____

Question: _____

Response: _____

Question: _____

Response: _____

Question: _____

Response: _____

Question: _____

Response: _____

Question: _____

Response: _____

Question: _____

Response: _____

Question: _____

Response: _____

Neurovascular Pathology

Question: _____

Response: _____

Question: _____

Response: _____

Question: _____

Response: _____

Question: _____

Response: _____

Question: _____

Response: _____

Question: _____

Response: _____

Question: _____

Response: _____

Question: _____

Response: _____

Question: _____

Response: _____

Question: _____

Response: _____

Question: _____

Response: _____

ACTIVITY 3   Range of Motion

Introduction

Range of motion (ROM) is the amount of motion available at a joint. The assessment of ROM should include active ROM (AROM), passive ROM (PROM), and resisted ROM (RROM) movements. Active movements, which are performed by the patient, are always evaluated first. The examiner should note the available ROM and any discomfort experienced by the patient. Passive movement performed by the examiner is assessed next. The quantity of this movement can be assessed with goniometry, and the quality is assessed by noting pain and the type of end-feel. ROM testing is then completed with the examiner providing resistance to the movement.

Assessing ROM with *goniometry,* which literally means "to measure angles," involves the use of a goniometer to measure the movement of the shafts of bones.

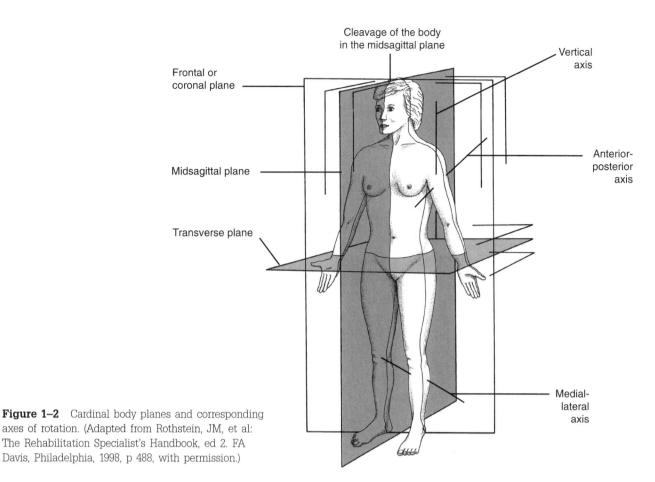

Cleavage of the body
in the midsagittal plane

Vertical
axis

Frontal or
coronal plane

Midsagittal plane

Transverse plane

Anterior-
posterior
axis

Medial-
lateral
axis

Figure 1–2   Cardinal body planes and corresponding
axes of rotation. (Adapted from Rothstein, JM, et al:
The Rehabilitation Specialist's Handbook, ed 2. FA
Davis, Philadelphia, 1998, p 488, with permission.)

This movement is termed *osteokinematics*. The fulcrum of the goniometer is placed
on the axis of rotation of the joint. To measure ROM, identify the cardinal plane of
movement. Each cardinal plane has a corresponding axis of rotation (Fig. 1–2), as
follows:

Cardinal Plane	Corresponding Axis of Rotation
Sagittal	Medial-lateral
Frontal	Anterior-posterior
Transverse	Vertical

The fulcrum of the goniometer is aligned with the corresponding axis of rotation of the joint being assessed. The stationary arm is aligned over the proximal segment of the joint. The movement arm is aligned over the distal segment. The 0- to
180-degree measuring system is recommended. With this system, all joints are considered to be at 0 degrees in the anatomical position. Movement in any direction is
described toward 180 degrees. The joint is measured in extension and then moved
into flexion. Care is needed to stabilize the joint to prevent unwanted movement.
The moveable arm of the goniometer is then moved to correspond with the new position of the distal shaft, and a measurement is taken (Fig. 1–3).

Instructions ➤   Assess PROM for the movements listed on the following page. Compare the results
bilaterally and to the normal ROMs reported in your textbook.

	Range of Motion (Degrees)		
	Right	**Left**	**Normal**
ANKLE			
Dorsiflexion			
Plantar flexion			
SUBTALAR JOINT			
Inversion			
Eversion			
KNEE			
Flexion			
Extension			
Internal rotation with knee flexed			
External rotation with knee flexed			
HIP			
Flexion with knee extended			
Flexion with knee flexed			
Extension			
Abduction			
Adduction			
Internal rotation			
External rotation			
SHOULDER			
Flexion			
Extension			
Abduction			
Adduction			
Internal rotation			
External rotation			
ELBOW			
Flexion			
Extension			
Pronation			
Supination			
WRIST			
Flexion			
Extension			
Ulnar deviation			
Radial deviation			

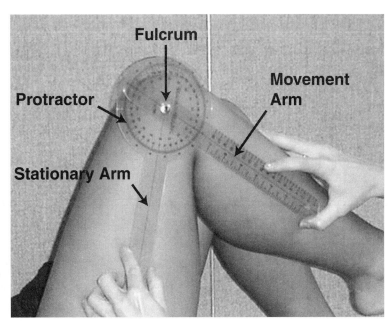

Figure 1–3   Using a goniometer to measure a joint's range of motion. (From Starkey, C, and Ryan, J: Evaluation of Orthopedic and Athletic Injuries, ed 2. FA Davis, Philadelphia, 2002, with permission.)

ACTIVITY 4   Resisted Range of Motion

Introduction

Resisted ROM (RROM) can be used to assess muscle function. After a thorough assessment, the muscle should be graded using the following chart:

Grade	Number	%	Description
Zero	0	0	No contraction
Trace	1	10	Slight contraction, unable to produce motion
Poor	2	25	Complete ROM when gravity eliminated
Fair	3	50	Complete ROM against resistance of gravity
Good	4	75	Complete ROM against gravity plus moderate resistance
Normal	5	100	Complete ROM against gravity plus maximum resistance

To complete this assessment, a number of factors, such as patient positioning, joint stabilization, mechanical advantage, and muscle actions, must be considered.

Instructions ➤   Please review the corresponding sections in your textbook before completing this exercise. Position your patient as indicated, and stabilize the joint to prevent unwanted movement. Patient positioning for the hip includes both gravity-dependent and gravity-eliminated positions to distinguish between muscle function of grade 2 and that of grade 3. Only gravity-dependent positions used to identify grades 4 and 5 are included for the other joints.

Instruct your patient to perform the following series of muscular movements: active, passive, and resisted. Resisted movements should include concentric, eccentric, and isometric muscle actions. Identify prime movers as you complete the assessment.

Joint and Range of Motion	Position	Prime Movers
HIP		
Flexion	Without gravity—side-lying	
	With gravity—short sitting	
Extension	Without gravity—side-lying	
	With gravity—lying prone	
Abduction	Without gravity—long sitting	
	With gravity—side-lying	
	Resistive—short sitting	
Adduction	Without gravity—long sitting	
	With gravity—side-lying	
	Resistive—short sitting	
Internal rotation	Without gravity—long sitting	
	With gravity—short sitting	
External rotation*	Without gravity—long sitting	
	With gravity—short sitting	
ANKLE		
Dorsiflexion	Supine with foot and ankle extending beyond table	
Plantar flexion	Supine with foot and ankle extending beyond table	
Inversion	Supine with foot and ankle extending beyond table	
Eversion	Supine with foot and ankle extending beyond table	
KNEE		
Flexion	Prone with patella and lower leg extending beyond table	
Extension	Short sitting	
Internal rotation	Short sitting	
External rotation	Short sitting	
SHOULDER		
Flexion	Short sitting, with examiner along side	
Extension	Lying prone	
Abduction	Short sitting with examiner behind	

*Moving leg medially is actually external rotation.

Joint and Range of Motion	Position	Prime Movers
Horizontal adduction	Lying supine with elbow flexed to 90 degrees	
Internal rotation	Lying prone with 90 degrees shoulder abduction and elbow flexion	
External rotation	Lying prone with 90 degrees shoulder abduction and elbow flexion	
ELBOW		
Flexion	Short sitting with examiner in front	
Extension	Lying prone with 90 degrees shoulder abduction	
Pronation	Short sitting, patient holding short bar	
Supination	Short sitting, patient holding short bar	
WRIST		
Flexion	Short sitting with forearm supported on table	
Extension	Short sitting with forearm supported on table	
Ulnar deviation	Short sitting with forearm supported on table	
Radial deviation	Short sitting with forearm supported on table	

ACTIVITY 5   Two-Joint Muscles to Aid in Assessing Muscle Function

Introduction

Several muscles cross two joints and have an action on each joint. These muscles are called two-joint muscles. If movement is caused by two muscles, where one is a prime mover for only the intended movement, and the other is a two-joint muscle that is a prime mover for an additional movement, tests can be performed to determine which muscle is injured. Two tests using hip flexion as an example are provided.

EXAMPLE: Hip flexion involving the iliopsoas and rectus femoris (RF) muscles

Resisted hip flexion causes pain, and strength is decreased; therefore either the iliopsoas or RF is injured. To distinguish which muscle is injured, do the following:

1. Resisted knee extension:

   —If pain and decreased strength occur, the RF muscle is injured.

   —If no pain occurs in conjunction with decreased strength, the iliopsoas muscle is injured.

2. First test hip flexion with the knee flexed, then extend the knee to shorten the RF before completing resisted hip flexion. By shortening the RF at the knee, it will contribute less to hip flexion.

   —If the pain and strength difference increase, the iliopsoas muscle is affected.

   —If the pain and strength difference decrease, the RF muscle is affected.

Instructions ➤ Identify the two-joint muscles for each of the following anatomical movements. Discuss with your partner how these muscles can be used in the assessment. Record your plan in the space provided.

Plantar flexion _____

Knee flexion _____

Knee extension _____

Hip flexion _____

Hip extension _____

Shoulder flexion _____

Elbow flexion _____

Elbow extension _____

ACTIVITY 6   RROM for Specific Muscles

Introduction

Often, knowing the anatomical movement affected by muscular injury is sufficient to adequately assess the injury and plan appropriate rehabilitation. In such cases, the assessment described previously is all that is necessary. However, identifying the individual muscle being affected is sometimes helpful in planning appropriate rehabilitation. Noting the location of pain during manual muscle testing may provide information for identifying the specific muscle involved. In some cases, such as when differentiating between the gastrocnemius and the soleus, isolating a muscle during the test is a necessary step.

Instructions ➤ Complete a manual muscle test that will isolate each of the following muscles:

Soleus _____

Gastrocnemius _____

Sartorius _____

Rectus femoris _____

Iliopsoas _____

Gluteus maximus _____

Hamstrings _____

Pectoralis major _____

Brachialis _____

Biceps brachii _____

Anterior deltoid _____

Triceps brachii _____

Posterior deltoid _____

ACTIVITY 7   Injury Nomenclature and Techniques

Definitions

Define the following terminology related to injury and assessment:

Tenosynovitis _____

Myositis ossificans _____

Apprehension response _____

Synovitis _____

Osteochondritis dissecans _____

Wolff's law _____

Exostosis _____

Apophysitis _____

Neurotmesis _____

Reflex sympathetic dystrophy _____

Errors in Terminology Usage

This activity is designed to improve your knowledge of basic injury terminology. Look through newspaper articles for inaccuracies in terminology (e.g., "strained a ligament in his knee"). Share any transgressions with the class.

Medical vs. Layperson Terminology

Place the letter of the appropriate medical term in the right-hand column next to the correct layperson's term or phrase listed in the left-hand column. Keep in mind that the terms on the right may be used once or not at all.

_____	1. "I pulled a muscle."	A. Exostosis
_____	2. "I separated my shoulder."	B. Sprain
_____	3. "My shoulder went out."	C. Fracture
_____	4. "I have water on my knee."	D. Effusion
_____	5. "I tore a ligament."	E. Swelling
_____	6. "My leg turned black and blue."	F. Subluxation
_____	7. "I have a calcium deposit in my leg."	G. Ecchymosis
_____	8. "I have bone chips in my elbow."	H. Hematoma

_____ 9. "I have a heel spur."

_____ 10. "I have a stinger."

I. Myositis ossificans

J. Osteochondritis dissecans

K. Strain

L. Neuropraxia

Matching exercise from Brown, S: Instructor's Guide for Starkey and Ryan's Evaluation of Orthopedic and Athletic Injuries. FA Davis, Philadelphia, 1997, p 12, with permission.

Imaging Techniques

Use available resources to collect hard copies of different imaging techniques (e.g., x-ray, magnetic resonance imaging). Share these with the class and try to identify the pathological condition. If time permits, take a field trip to a local imaging center so that you can see what the machines actually look like and get a description of how the process occurs (e.g., duration, any necessary injections, positioning).

ANSWER KEY

Activity 7

1. K
2. B
3. F
4. D
5. B
6. G
7. I
8. J
9. A
10. L

Chapter 2

Assessing the Foot, Ankle, and Lower Leg

CHAPTER OUTLINE

ACTIVITY 1   History

Instructions ➤ Have your partner select a common acute injury from the body part that you are studying. Ask a series of questions in an attempt to narrow the injury possibilities and guide the assessment. Your partner should provide the answers that would be likely from an athlete with this injury. Record all questions and responses, and discuss your conclusions with your partner and your instructor. Repeat the process using a chronic injury.

Acute Injury

Question: _____

Response: _____

Question: _____

Response: _____

Question: _____

Response: _____

Question: _____

Response: _____

Question: _____

Response: _____

Question: _____

Response: _____

Question: _____

Response: _____

Question: _____

Response: _____

Question: _____

Response: _____

Question: _____

Response: _____

Question: _____

Response: _____

Question: _____

Response: _____

Chronic Injury

Question: _____

Response: _____

Question: _____

Response: _____

Question: _____

Response: _____

Question: _____

Response: _____

Question: _____

Response: _____

Question: _____

Response: _____

Question: _____

Response: _____

Question: _____

Response: _____

Question: _____

Response: _____

Question: _____

Response: _____

Question: _____

Response: _____

Question: _____

Response: _____

ACTIVITY 2   Inspection

Instructions ➤ Define the deformities, abnormalities, and conditions listed here. Inspect your partner's lower extremity to identify each condition. Inspect other students until each of the conditions has been found. If a condition is not found within the class population, find a photograph of the deformity in your textbook.

Abnormal Feet

Pronation (calcaneovalgus or hindfoot valgus) _____

Supination (calcaneovarus or hindfoot varus) _____

Pes cavus _____

Pes planus (structural vs. flexible/supple) _____

Morton's toe _____

Foot Deformities and Conditions

Claw toes _____

Mallet toes _____

Hammer toes _____

Bunions (hallux valgus) _____

Bunionettes _____

Plantar warts _____

Corns—hard and soft _____

Pump bump (Haglund's deformity) _____

Instructions ➤ Obtaining quantitative measurements may be necessary to directly identify conditions or identify predisposing factors important in the overall assessment. Complete the following measurements on your partner, and compare the measurements bilaterally when appropriate. Compare these measurements with those of other class-

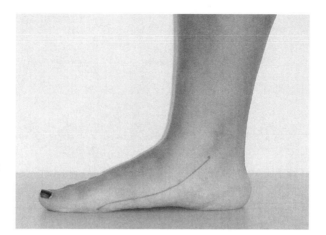

Figure 2–1   Feiss' line. (From Starkey, C, and Ryan, J: Evaluation of Orthopedic and Athletic Injuries, ed 2. FA Davis, Philadelphia, 2002, with permission.)

mates and against normal values. If pathological values are found, discuss the implications for orthopedic injury and possible methods of intervention.

■ Feiss' line (Fig. 2–1)
■ Navicular drop test

Record the distance of drop for the following:

Partner's right foot   _____

Partner's left foot   _____

Classmate's right foot   _____

Classmate's left foot   _____

ACTIVITY 3   Palpation

Bony Palpation

Instructions ➤   Review the sections on the bony anatomy of the foot, ankle, and lower leg in your textbook before completing this exercise. Begin by locating each bony landmark listed on Fig. 2–2, using the help of your textbook when needed. Develop a systematic approach so that no important structures are missed. Complete the remainder of the assignment after taking a break.

Without the aid of your textbook or skeleton, locate each bony landmark on your partner. When you have found the landmark, mark its location with a small sticker and place a check next to the landmark listed here. Use available resources (e.g., textbook, skeleton, instructor) to check the accuracy of your palpation markers.

Medial Aspect

☐ First metatarsal-phalangeal joint
☐ First metatarsal
☐ First cuneiform
☐ Navicular tubercle
☐ Sustentaculum tali
☐ Medial malleolus
☐ Talus

Lateral and Medial Views

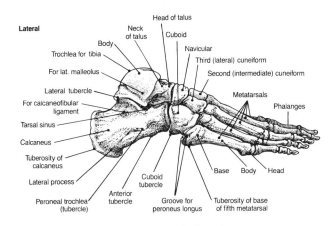

Figure 2–2 Anatomy of the foot showing prominent bony landmarks and sites of ligamentous and muscular attachments. (From Rothstein, JM, Roy, SH, and Wolf, SL: The Rehabilitation Specialist's Handbook, ed 2. FA Davis, Philadelphia, 1998, p 93, with permission.)

Lateral Aspect

☐ Fifth metatarsal-phalangeal joint
☐ Styloid process (tubercle) of fifth metatarsal
☐ Cuboid
☐ Peroneal tubercle
☐ Lateral malleolus

Dorsal Aspect

☐ Phalanges
☐ Metatarsals
☐ Cuneiforms
☐ Sinus tarsi

Plantar Aspect

☐ Sesamoid bones
☐ Metatarsal heads
☐ Medial calcaneal tubercle
☐ Retrocalcaneal apophysis

Soft Tissue Palpation

Instructions ➤ Review the sections on soft tissue anatomy of the foot, ankle, and lower leg in your textbook before completing this exercise. Begin by locating each structure in a figure in your textbook. Develop a systematic approach so that no important structures are missed. Complete the remainder of the assignment after taking a break.

Without the aid of your textbook or skeleton, locate each structure on your partner. When you have found the landmark, mark its location with a small sticker and place a check next to the landmark listed here. For larger or lengthy structures, mark a prominent portion. Use available resources (e.g., textbook, skeleton, instructor) to check the accuracy of your palpation markers.

Medial Aspect

☐ Deltoid ligament
☐ Spring ligament
☐ Flexor hallucis longus
☐ Flexor digitorum longus
☐ Tibialis posterior

Lateral Aspect

☐ Anterior talofibular (ATF) ligament
☐ Posterior talofibular (PTF) ligament
☐ Calcaneofibular ligament
☐ Peroneus brevis
☐ Peroneal retinaculum

Dorsal Aspect

☐ Anterior tibiofibular ligament
☐ Tibialis anterior
☐ Extensor hallucis longus
☐ Extensor digitorum longus
☐ Extensor digitorum brevis
☐ Extensor retinaculum

Plantar Aspect

☐ Achilles tendon
☐ Plantar fascia

ACTIVITY 4   Range-of-Motion Tests

Instructions ➤ Ask your patient to complete active range of motion (AROM) for the movements listed here. Note the available range of motion (ROM) and any discomfort.

Passive Range of Motion

After observing AROM, assess passive range of motion (PROM) for the movements listed on page 24. Compare the results bilaterally and with the normal ROMs reported in your textbook.

	Range of Motion (Degrees)		
	Right	Left	Normal
ANKLE			
Dorsiflexion	_____	_____	_____
Plantar flexion	_____	_____	_____
SUBTALAR JOINT			
Inversion	_____	_____	_____
Eversion	_____	_____	_____

End-feels

PROM should include an assessment of end-feels. Provide a force at the end of the PROM and note the sensation. Record the physiological end-feel for the movement indicated, and note whether a pathological end-feel is present.

	Physiological End-feel	Pathological End-feel (If Present)
ANKLE		
Dorsiflexion	_____	_____
Plantar flexion	_____	_____
SUBTALAR JOINT		
Inversion	_____	_____
Eversion	_____	_____

Resisted Range of Motion

Complete resisted range of motion (RROM) for the movements listed here. Position your patient as indicated, and stabilize the joint to prevent unwanted movement. Resistive movements should include concentric, eccentric, and isometric muscle actions. Identify prime movers as you complete the assessment.

Range of Motion and Position	Movements (Concentric, Eccentric, and Isometric)	Prime Movers
ANKLE		
Dorsiflexion—supine with foot and ankle extending beyond table	_____	_____
Plantar flexion—supine with foot and ankle extending beyond table	_____	_____
SUBTALAR JOINT		
Inversion—supine with foot and ankle extending beyond table	_____	_____
Eversion—supine with foot and ankle extending beyond table	_____	_____

ACTIVITY 5   Joint Stability Tests

Introduction

Injury to ligaments supporting a joint can be identified through stability tests. During these stability tests, *laxity,* or the amount of movement allowed by a joint's capsule and ligaments, is compared bilaterally. In addition, the *end-feel,* or sensation felt by the examiner at the limit of the stability test, is noted. Generally speaking, the end-feel during a stability test of a healthy joint is firm and definite, whereas the end-feel of an injured joint is soft and indefinite.

Instructions ➤ Provide the name for the stability test designed to test the given ligament, and then perform each test using classmates as patients. If more than one blank is included, provide alternative tests. Inherent variability of laxity exists among the healthy population. Complete the stability tests on several subjects until you have identified classmates with different grades of laxity. When two classmates with differences in laxity have been identified, you can perform the stability tests to get a better feel for a positive sign of laxity. In an actual injury assessment, this comparison would be made bilaterally.

After completing the assignment, discuss with your partner any joint position changes that should be performed before the stability test (e.g., flexion, rotation). Discuss the purpose for these changes in joint position.

Ankle Ligaments	Stability Tests
Calcaneofibular ligament	_____
Deltoid ligament	_____
	_____
Anterior talofibular ligament (ATF)	_____
Anterior and posterior tibiofibular ligaments	_____
	_____

ACTIVITY 6   Special Tests

Introduction

Certain specific injuries and conditions, such as a ruptured Achilles tendon, require special tests that do not fit into the other assessment categories. Often, these tests are designed to stress a specific structure through scripted movements.

Instructions ➤ Provide the name for or describe (if there is no specific name) the special test or tests that may be used to identify the injuries and conditions listed here. Complete the special tests using your partner as the injured athlete. Describe a positive sign, and record this information in the space provided. If more than one blank is included, provide alternative tests.

Injury/Condition	Special Test	Positive Sign
Achilles tendon rupture	_____	_____
Supple pes planus	_____	_____

ACTIVITY 7 Neurologic Tests

Instructions ➤ Complete a thorough neurologic assessment for the foot and toes by completing the tests outlined in the following chart. Include dermatome, myotome, and reflex testing.

Nerve Root	Dermatome	Sensory Nerve	Myotome	Motor Nerve	Reflex
L4	Medial leg; first toe	Saphenous	Dorsiflexion	Deep peroneal	Patellar
L5	Anterior leg; second to fourth toes	Peroneal	Toe extension	Deep peroneal	Patellar
S1	Lateral leg/foot; Achilles	Peroneal	Plantar flexion	Tibial	Achilles
S2	Posterior leg	Femoral cutaneous	None	Lateral plantar	Achilles

ACTIVITY 8 Skill Integration: Foot and Toe

Scenario A female distance runner comes to you in the athletic training room complaining of right foot pain that has gotten progressively worse over the past month. Demonstrate and explain your assessment of this injury. The model will not respond to your questions but will perform any actions that you request.

Optional: You have _____ minutes to complete your evaluation.

Evaluation

Name: _____   *Date:* _____

History

Establishes any specific mechanism of injury	YES	☐	NO	☐
Establishes prior history of injury to either foot	YES	☐	NO	☐
Establishes location of pain	YES	☐	NO	☐
Establishes type of pain	YES	☐	NO	☐
Establishes treatment (if any) since injury	YES	☐	NO	☐
Establishes changes in training pattern (e.g., surface)	YES	☐	NO	☐
Establishes current training pattern	YES	☐	NO	☐
Establishes progression of symptoms	YES	☐	NO	☐
Establishes presence or absence of neurologic symptoms	YES	☐	NO	☐
Establishes presence or absence of pain elsewhere on the body	YES	☐	NO	☐

Inspection

Inspects for the following:

Swelling	YES	☐	NO	☐
Discoloration	YES	☐	NO	☐
Deformity (e.g., claw toes, hallux valgus)	YES	☐	NO	☐
Gait abnormalities	YES	☐	NO	☐
Skin changes (e.g., calluses, corns)	YES	☐	NO	☐
Foot type (supinated, pronated, neutral)	YES	☐	NO	☐
Foot/calcaneal alignment (in standing)	YES	☐	NO	☐
Foot/calcaneal alignment (prone; subtalar neutral)	YES	☐	NO	☐
Inspects running shoes for abnormal wear patterns	YES	☐	NO	☐
Compares inspected areas bilaterally	YES	☐	NO	☐

(Must expose both feet to get credit for this.)

Palpation

Palpates for presence of the following:

Point tenderness	YES	☐	NO	☐
Swelling	YES	☐	NO	☐
Temperature change	YES	☐	NO	☐
Deformity	YES	☐	NO	☐
Performs all palpation bilaterally (or states would do so)	YES	☐	NO	☐

Palpates bony and ligamentous structures:

Phalanges (first through fifth digits)	YES	☐	NO	☐
Metatarsal-phalangeal joints (first through fifth)	YES	☐	NO	☐
Sesamoids	YES	☐	NO	☐
Metatarsals (first through fifth)	YES	☐	NO	☐
Styloid process (fifth metatarsal)	YES	☐	NO	☐

(Continued)

Cuboid .... YES ☐ NO ☐

Talar dome .... YES ☐ NO ☐

Calcaneus (medial tubercle, posterior flair) .... YES ☐ NO ☐

Talar head .... YES ☐ NO ☐

Spring ligament .... YES ☐ NO ☐

Navicular .... YES ☐ NO ☐

Midtarsal articulations .... YES ☐ NO ☐

Cuneiforms .... YES ☐ NO ☐

Palpates other soft tissues:

Flexor hallucis longus (FHL) tendon .... YES ☐ NO ☐

Flexor digitorum longus (FDL) tendon .... YES ☐ NO ☐

Posterior tibialis tendon .... YES ☐ NO ☐

Plantar fascia .... YES ☐ NO ☐

Tibialis anterior muscle and tendon .... YES ☐ NO ☐

Extensor hallucis longus (EHL) tendon .... YES ☐ NO ☐

Extensor digitorum longus (EDL) tendon .... YES ☐ NO ☐

Extensor digitorum brevis muscle .... YES ☐ NO ☐

Peroneal tendons .... YES ☐ NO ☐

Range-of-Motion Testing

Response is incorrect if all motions (metatarsal-phalangeal joint flexion and extension) are not included. Action must be performed correctly (i.e., proper hand placement, adequate resistance). (Ankle motions can be included at the discretion of the instructor.)

Evaluates AROM .... YES ☐ NO ☐

Evaluates PROM .... YES ☐ NO ☐

Evaluates RROM (first separate from second through fifth) .... YES ☐ NO ☐

Performs all ROM bilaterally (or states would do so) .... YES ☐ NO ☐

Ligamentous and Capsular Testing

Response is incorrect if test is not performed correctly (i.e., proper hand placement, appropriate direction and amount of stress).

Valgus stress testing of metatarsal-phalangeal and interphalangeal joints .... YES ☐ NO ☐

Varus stress testing of metatarsal-phalangeal and interphalangeal joints .... YES ☐ NO ☐

Proximal intermetatarsal joints (glide between metatarsal heads) .... YES ☐ NO ☐

Intermetatarsal glide .... YES ☐ NO ☐

Performs all tests bilaterally .... YES ☐ NO ☐

Special Tests

Response is incorrect if test is not performed correctly (i.e., proper hand positioning, appropriate direction and amount of stress).

Assessment of extent of pes planus (i.e., Feiss' line, navicular drop test, non–weight bearing to weight bearing) .... YES ☐ NO ☐

Performs test bilaterally .... YES ☐ NO ☐

Presentation

Performs evaluation in a confident, professional manner .... YES ☐   NO ☐

Performs evaluation in a logical sequence .... YES ☐   NO ☐

Performs evaluation within allotted time .... YES ☐   NO ☐

TOTAL: _____ / _____

Evaluator: _____

ACTIVITY 9   Skill Integration: Ankle

Scenario   A wrestler comes to you in the athletic training room complaining of right ankle pain after "twisting" his ankle yesterday during practice. Demonstrate and explain your assessment of this injury. The model will not respond to your questions but will perform any actions that you request.

Optional: You have _____ minutes to complete your evaluation.

Evaluation

Name: _____ Date: _____

History

Establishes mechanism of injury	YES	☐	NO	☐
Establishes location of pain	YES	☐	NO	☐
Establishes type of pain	YES	☐	NO	☐
Establishes treatment (if any) since injury	YES	☐	NO	☐
Asks if "pop" was felt or heard	YES	☐	NO	☐
Establishes prior history of injury to either ankle	YES	☐	NO	☐
Establishes presence or absence of pain elsewhere in the body	YES	☐	NO	☐

Inspection

Inspects for the following:

Swelling	YES	☐	NO	☐
Discoloration	YES	☐	NO	☐
Deformity	YES	☐	NO	☐
Gait	YES	☐	NO	☐
States that observation occurs bilaterally	YES	☐	NO	☐

(Must expose both feet to get credit for this.)

Palpation

Palpates for presence of the following:

Point tenderness	YES	☐	NO	☐
Swelling	YES	☐	NO	☐
Temperature change	YES	☐	NO	☐
Deformity	YES	☐	NO	☐
Performs all palpation bilaterally (or states would do so)	YES	☐	NO	☐

Palpates bony and ligamentous structures:

Distal tibia	YES	☐	NO	☐
Entire fibula	YES	☐	NO	☐
Base of fifth metatarsal	YES	☐	NO	☐
Calcaneus	YES	☐	NO	☐
Navicular	YES	☐	NO	☐
Cuboid	YES	☐	NO	☐
Dome of talus	YES	☐	NO	☐
Cuneiforms	YES	☐	NO	☐
Anterior talofibular (ATF) ligament	YES	☐	NO	☐
Calcaneofibular (CF) ligament	YES	☐	NO	☐
Posterior talofibular (PTF) ligament	YES	☐	NO	☐
Deltoid ligament	YES	☐	NO	☐
Midtarsal articulations	YES	☐	NO	☐

Tibia-fibula ligaments and articulation ....YES ☐   NO ☐

Palpates other soft tissue:

Extensor digitorum brevis ....YES ☐   NO ☐

Peroneal tendons ....YES ☐   NO ☐

Anterior tibialis tendon ....YES ☐   NO ☐

Long toe flexor tendons ....YES ☐   NO ☐

Long toe extensor tendons ....YES ☐   NO ☐

Range-of-Motion Testing

Response is incorrect if all motions (dorsiflexion, plantar flexion, inversion, and eversion) are not included. Action must be performed correctly (i.e., proper hand placement, adequate resistance, elimination of substituting movements).

Evaluates AROM ....YES ☐   NO ☐

Evaluates PROM ....YES ☐   NO ☐

Evaluates RROM ....YES ☐   NO ☐

Performs all ROM bilaterally (or states would do so) ....YES ☐   NO ☐

Ligamentous and Capsular Testing

Response is incorrect if test is not performed correctly (i.e., proper hand placement, appropriate direction and amount of stress).

Performs anterior drawer test ....YES ☐   NO ☐

Performs talar tilt test (inversion stress) ....YES ☐   NO ☐

Performs talar tilt test (eversion stress) ....YES ☐   NO ☐

Performs Kleiger test ....YES ☐   NO ☐

Performs tests bilaterally (or states would do so) ....YES ☐   NO ☐

Special Tests

Response is incorrect if test is not performed correctly (i.e., proper hand positioning, appropriate direction and amount of stress).

Bump test (rule out fracture) ....YES ☐   NO ☐

Squeeze test (mortise disruption) ....YES ☐   NO ☐

Thompson test ....YES ☐   NO ☐

Performs tests bilaterally (or states would do so) ....YES ☐   NO ☐

Presentation

Performs evaluation in a confident, professional manner ....YES ☐   NO ☐

Performs evaluation in a logical sequence ....YES ☐   NO ☐

Performs evaluation within allotted time ....YES ☐   NO ☐

TOTAL: _____ / _____

Evaluator: _____

Comments: _____

ACTIVITY 10   Skill Integration: Lower Leg

Scenario   A distance runner who is a college junior comes to you complaining of left lower leg pain that has gotten progressively worse over the past 3 weeks. Demonstrate and explain your assessment of this injury. The model will not respond to your questions but will perform any actions that you request.

Optional: You have _____ minutes to complete your evaluation.

Evaluation

Name: _____   Date: _____

History

Establishes any mechanism of injury	YES	☐	NO	☐
Establishes prior history	YES	☐	NO	☐
Establishes location of pain	YES	☐	NO	☐
Establishes type of pain	YES	☐	NO	☐
Establishes pain pattern (i.e., at rest? in A.M.?)	YES	☐	NO	☐
Establishes workout pattern (i.e., recent increase in mileage, hills)	YES	☐	NO	☐
Establishes age/type of running shoe	YES	☐	NO	☐
Establishes presence/absence of neurologic symptoms	YES	☐	NO	☐

Inspection

Inspects for the following:

Swelling	YES	☐	NO	☐
Gait	YES	☐	NO	☐
Atrophy	YES	☐	NO	☐
Discoloration (glossiness)	YES	☐	NO	☐
Foot type (supinated, pronated, neutral)	YES	☐	NO	☐
Foot/calcaneal alignment (in standing)	YES	☐	NO	☐
Foot/calcaneal alignment (prone; subtalar neutral)	YES	☐	NO	☐
States that observation occurs bilaterally	YES	☐	NO	☐
Inspects shoes and/or soles of feet for wear/callous pattern	YES	☐	NO	☐

Palpation

Palpates for presence of the following:

Point tenderness	YES	☐	NO	☐
Temperature change	YES	☐	NO	☐
Rigidity	YES	☐	NO	☐
Swelling	YES	☐	NO	☐
Deformity	YES	☐	NO	☐
Performs all palpation bilaterally (or states would do so)	YES	☐	NO	☐

Palpates bony and ligamentous structures:

Tibia	YES	☐	NO	☐
Fibula	YES	☐	NO	☐

Palpates other soft tissue:

Anterior tibialis	YES	☐	NO	☐
Peroneals	YES	☐	NO	☐
Gastrocnemius/soleus/Achilles tendon	YES	☐	NO	☐

(Continued)

Range-of-Motion Testing

Response is incorrect if all motions (dorsiflexion, plantar flexion, inversion, eversion, and toe flexion/extension [resisted only]) are not included. Action must be performed correctly (i.e., proper hand placement, adequate resistance, elimination of substituting movements).

Evaluates AROM (ankle dorsiflexion, plantar flexion, eversion, inversion) ....YES ☐   NO ☐

Evaluates PROM (ankle dorsiflexion, plantar flexion, eversion, inversion) ....YES ☐   NO ☐

Evaluates PROM (ankle dorsiflexion, plantar flexion, eversion, inversion,
toe flexion/extension) ....YES ☐   NO ☐

Special Tests

Response is incorrect if test is not performed correctly (i.e., proper hand position, appropriate direction and amount of stress).

Bump test ....YES ☐   NO ☐

Squeeze test ....YES ☐   NO ☐

Neurovascular Assessment

Evaluates distal sensation (first web space) ....YES ☐   NO ☐

Evaluates distal pulse (dorsal pedal) ....YES ☐   NO ☐

Presentation

Performs evaluation in a confident, professional manner ....YES ☐   NO ☐

Performs evaluation in a logical sequence ....YES ☐   NO ☐

Performs evaluation within allotted time ....YES ☐   NO ☐

TOTAL: _____ / _____

Evaluator: _____

ACTIVITY 11 Practical Questions

Instructions ➤ After reading the chapter in your textbook dealing with the foot, ankle, and lower leg, and completing the corresponding activities, complete the following questions using your lab partner as the patient. The performance evaluation sheets that follow can be used by your instructor to grade the quality of your response to each question.

1. Complete the bony palpation of the foot. Name the bones of the foot, bony prominence, sites affected by athletic injuries and conditions, and articulations as you palpate them.

2. Name the three arches of the foot. Show their location on your subject by palpating them. Identify the bony margins and supporting structures of each arch.

3. Your athlete is complaining of pain on the posterior, plantar surface of the foot. Identify a common injury that you might suspect, and complete the following: history (three most important questions) and palpation (what you are looking for). Identify any anatomical abnormalities that may predispose your athlete to this condition.

4. Perform all stability tests for the ankle complex. For each test, include the name, description, and positive signs.

5. Assess AROM at the ankle complex. Include normal values, and identify how you can tell whether ROM is abnormal. After completing the active move-

ments, assess PROM and identify the physiological end-feel for each anatomical movement.

6. Complete a thorough assessment of RROM at the ankle. Include a prime mover for each anatomical movement.

7. Define *supination* and *pronation*. Complete two tests for hyperpronation. Include positive signs in your answer.

PERFORMANCE EVALUATION SHEETS

1. *Complete the bony palpation of the foot. Name the bones of the foot, bony prominence, sites affected by athletic injuries and conditions, and articulations as you palpate them.*

Performance evaluation calcaneofibular

	Name	Palpation	Associated Injuries
Phalanges	_____	_____	
Metatarsals	_____	_____	_____
Styloid process	_____	_____	
Base of fifth	_____	_____	_____
Cuneiforms	_____	_____	
Cuboid	_____	_____	
Navicular	_____	_____	
Tubercle	_____	_____	
Talus	_____	_____	
Calcaneus			
Medial tubercle	_____	_____	_____
Retrocalcaneal apophysis	_____	_____	_____
Sustentaculum tali	_____	_____	
Peroneal tubercle	_____	_____	
Sinus tarsi	_____	_____	
Distal interphalangeal joints	_____	_____	_____
Proximal interphalangeal joints	_____	_____	_____
Metatarsal-phalangeal joints	_____	_____	
First and fifth	_____	_____	_____
Sesamoids	_____	_____	_____
Systematic approach	_____		
Bilateral comparison	_____		

(Continued)

2. *Name the three arches of the foot. Show their location on your subject by palpating them. Identify the bony margins and supporting structures of each arch.*

Performance evaluation

	Name	**Location (Palpation)**
1. Medial longitudinal arch	_____	_____
2. Lateral longitudinal arch	_____	_____
3. Transverse metatarsal arch	_____	_____

BONY MARGINS

1. Calcaneus to distal head of first metatarsal _____
2. Calcaneus to distal head of fifth metatarsal _____
3. Across the distal heads of the five metatarsals _____

SUPPORTING STRUCTURES

1. Spring ligament _____

Plantar fascia _____

2. Plantar fascia _____

3. Intermetatarsal ligaments _____

3. *Your athlete is complaining of pain on the posterior, plantar surface of the foot. Identify a common injury that you might suspect, and complete the following: history (three most important questions) and palpation (what you are looking for). Identify any anatomical abnormalities that may predispose your athlete to this condition.*

Performance evaluation

INJURY

Plantar fasciitis _____

Heel spur _____

HISTORY

Onset of symptoms (mechanism) _____

Previous injury _____

Type of pain _____

Location of pain _____

What worsens or relieves pain _____

What time of day is most painful _____

PALPATION

Medial calcaneal tubercle _____

Point tenderness _____

Bony exostosis _____

Crepitus _____

ABNORMALITIES

Pes cavus _____

Tight Achilles tendon _____

Bilateral comparison _____

4. *Perform all stability tests for the ankle complex. For each test include the name, description, and positive signs.*

Performance evaluation

	Ligament	Test	Description
Talar tilt (inversion)	(CF)	_____	_____
_____ Talar tilt (eversion)	(Deltoid)	_____	_____
_____ Kleiger test	(Deltoid)	_____	_____
_____ Anterior drawer	(ATF)	_____	_____

POSITIVE SIGN

_____ Pain _____ Laxity _____ Soft end-feel Bilateral comparison _____

5. *Assess AROM at the ankle complex. Include normal values, and identify how you can tell whether ROM is abnormal. After completing the active movements, assess PROM and identify the physiological end-feel for each anatomical movement.*

Performance evaluation

	Normal Values	Goniometer	Fulcrum	Arms
Plantar flexion	(50)	_____	_____	_____
Dorsiflexion	(20)	_____	_____	_____
Inversion	(20)	_____	_____	_____
Eversion	(5)	_____	_____	_____

PHYSIOLOGICAL END-FEEL

Plantar flexion _____

Dorsiflexion _____

Inversion _____

Eversion _____

Bilateral comparison _____

6. *Complete a thorough assessment of RROM at the ankle. Include a prime mover for each anatomical movement.*

Performance evaluation

	Test	Prime Mover
Plantar flexion	_____	_____
Dorsiflexion	_____	_____
Inversion	_____	_____
Eversion	_____	_____

(Continued)

Active _____   Resistive _____

Isometric/breaking point test _____   Concentric _____   Eccentric _____

Bilateral comparison _____

7. *Define* supination *and* pronation. *Complete two tests for hyperpronation. Include positive signs in your answer.*

Performance evaluation

Supination _____

Pronation _____

	Test	Description	Positive Sign
_____ Feiss' line	_____	_____	_____
_____ Navicular drop test	_____	_____	_____
Bilateral comparison	_____		

ANSWER KEY

Activity 4   End-feels

Dorsiflexion	Firm
Plantar flexion	Usually firm, sometimes hard
Inversion	Firm
Eversion	Hard or firm

Activity 5

Calcaneofibular ligament	Inversion stress test (talar tilt)
Deltoid ligament	Eversion stress test (talar tilt)
	Kleiger test
Anterior talofibular ligament (ATF)	Anterior drawer test
Anterior and posterior tibiofibular ligaments	Kleiger test
	Passive dorsiflexion

Activity 6

Achilles tendon rupture	Thompson test	No plantar flexion
Supple pes planus	Supple pes planus test	Longitudinal arch disappears with weight bearing

Chapter 3

Assessing the Knee

CHAPTER OUTLINE

Activity 1   History

Instructions ➤   Have your partner select a common acute injury from the body part that you are studying. Ask a series of questions in an attempt to narrow the injury possibilities and guide the assessment. Your partner should provide the answers that would be likely from an athlete who sustained this injury. Record all questions and responses, and discuss your conclusions with your partner and instructor. Repeat the process using a chronic injury.

Acute Injury

Question: _____

Response: _____

Question: _____

Response: _____

Question: _____

Response: _____

Question: _____

Response: _____

Question: _____

Response: _____

Question: _____

Response: _____

Question: _____

Response: _____

Question: _____

Response: _____

Question: _____

Response: _____

Question: _____

Response: _____

Chronic Injury

Question: _____

Response: _____

Question: _____

Response: _____

Question: _____

Response: _____

Question: _____

Response: _____

Question: _____

Response: _____

Question: _____

Response: _____

Question: _____

Response: _____

Question: _____

Response: _____

Question: _____

Response: _____

Question: _____

Response: _____

ACTIVITY 2   Inspection

Instructions ➤ Define the deformities, abnormalities, and conditions listed here. Inspect your partner's lower extremity to identify each condition. Inspect other students until each of the conditions has been found. If a condition is not found within the class population, find a photograph of the deformity in your textbook.

Genu valgum (less than 180 degrees)   ——————————————————

Genu varum (greater than 195 degrees) ——————————————————

Genu recurvatum   ——————————————————

Patella alta (camel sign)   ——————————————————

Patella baja   ——————————————————

Squinting patella   ——————————————————

Frog-eyed patella   ——————————————————

Anteversion of femoral neck
(less than 15 degrees)   ——————————————————

Retroversion of femoral neck
(greater than 15 degrees)   ——————————————————

Instructions ➤ Obtaining quantitative measurements may be necessary to directly identify conditions or to identify predisposing factors important in the overall assessment. Complete the following measurements on your partner, and compare the measurements bilaterally when appropriate. Compare these measurements with those of other classmates and with normal values. If pathological values are found, discuss the implications for orthopedic injury and possible methods of intervention.

Q Angle

The Q angle indicates the direction of pull of the quadriceps muscle group. It is the angle formed by the intersection of two lines:

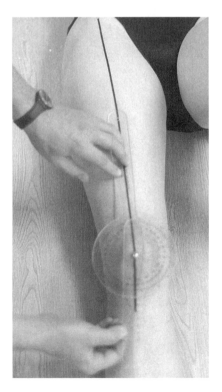

Figure 3–1 The Q angle. (From Starkey, C, and Ryan, J: Evaluation of Orthopedic and Athletic Injuries, ed 2. FA Davis, Philadelphia, 2001, p 250, with permission.)

■ Line from the anterior superior iliac spine (ASIS) through center of patella

■ Line through center of patella and tibial tuberosity (Fig. 3–1)

For males, the normal value is 13 degrees; for females, the normal value is 18 degrees. An angle of greater than 20 degrees may predispose a patient to patellar tracking injuries.

Record Q angles for the following:

Male classmate's right Q angle _____

Male classmate's left Q angle _____

Normal value for males _____

Female classmate's right Q angle _____

Female classmate's left Q angle _____

Normal value for females _____

Girth Measurements

Girth measurements for the knee can be used to identify atrophy or swelling (Fig. 3–2). Measurements should be made bilaterally over the following sites:

	Right Knee	Left Knee
6 inches above joint line	_____	_____
4 inches above joint line	_____	_____
2 inches above joint line	_____	_____
Joint line	_____	_____

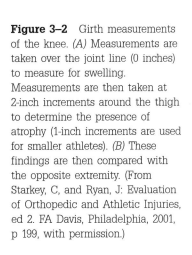

Figure 3–2 Girth measurements of the knee. *(A)* Measurements are taken over the joint line (0 inches) to measure for swelling. Measurements are then taken at 2-inch increments around the thigh to determine the presence of atrophy (1-inch increments are used for smaller athletes). *(B)* These findings are then compared with the opposite extremity. (From Starkey, C, and Ryan, J: Evaluation of Orthopedic and Athletic Injuries, ed 2. FA Davis, Philadelphia, 2001, p 199, with permission.)

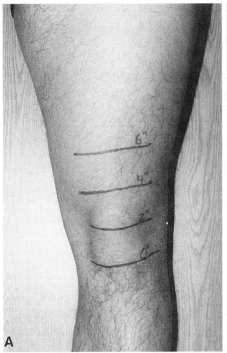

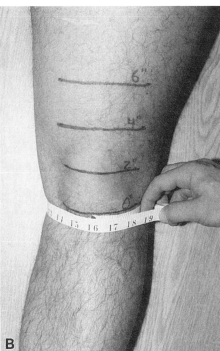

ACTIVITY 3   Palpation

Bony Palpation

Instructions ➤ Review the sections on bony anatomy in your textbook before completing this exercise. Begin by locating each bony landmark listed in Fig. 3–3 on a skeleton, using the help of your textbook when needed. Develop a systematic approach so that no important structures are missed. Complete the remainder of the assignment after taking a break.

Without the aid of your textbook or skeleton, locate each bony landmark on your partner. When you have found the landmark, mark its location with a small sticker and place a check next to the landmark listed here. Use available resources (e.g., textbook, skeleton, instructor) to check the accuracy of your palpation.

- ☐ Medial femoral condyle
- ☐ Lateral femoral condyle
- ☐ Medial tibial condyle
- ☐ Lateral tibial condyle
- ☐ Tibial tuberosity
- ☐ Pes anserinus
- ☐ Gerdy's tubercle
- ☐ Proximal head of fibula
- ☐ Superior patellar pole
- ☐ Inferior patellar pole
- ☐ Medial and lateral patellar borders

Soft Tissue Palpation

Instructions ➤ Review the sections on soft tissue anatomy of the knee in your textbook before completing this exercise (see Fig. 3–3). Begin by locating each structure in a figure in your textbook. Develop a systematic approach so that no important structures are missed. Complete the remainder of the assignment after taking a break.

Without the aid of your textbook or skeleton, locate each structure on your partner. When you have found the landmark, mark its location with a small sticker and place a check next to the landmark listed here. For lengthy or larger structures, mark a prominent portion. Use available resources (e.g., textbook, skeleton, instructor) to check the accuracy of your palpation markers.

Anterior Aspect

- ☐ Quadriceps tendon
- ☐ Patellar tendon
- ☐ Vastus medialis
- ☐ Vastus lateralis
- ☐ Rectus femoris

Posterior Aspect

- ☐ Popliteal fossa
- ☐ Medial and lateral head of gastrocnemius

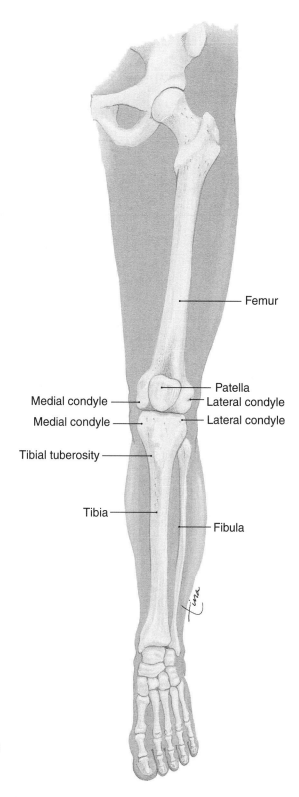

- Femur
- Patella
- Medial condyle
- Lateral condyle
- Medial condyle
- Lateral condyle
- Tibial tuberosity
- Tibia
- Fibula

Figure 3–3 Anatomy of the knee. (From Scanlon, VC, and Sanders, T: Understanding Human Structure and Function. FA Davis, Philadelphia, 1997, p 101, with permission.)

Medial Aspect

☐ Medial collateral ligament (MCL)
☐ Medial meniscus (joint line)
☐ Medial patellar retinaculum

Lateral Aspect

☐ Lateral collateral ligament (LCL)
☐ Lateral meniscus
☐ Lateral patellar retinaculum

Posteromedial Aspect

☐ Sartorius
☐ Gracilis
☐ Semitendinosus
☐ Semimembranosus

Posterolateral Aspect

☐ Iliotibial band
☐ Biceps femoris

ACTIVITY 4   Range-of-Motion Tests

Instructions ➤ Ask your patient to complete active range of motion (AROM) for the movements listed here. Note the available range of motion (ROM) and any discomfort.

Passive Range of Motion

After observing AROM, assess passive range of motion (PROM) for the following movements. Compare the results bilaterally and with the normal ROMs reported in your textbook.

	Range of Motion (Degrees)		
	Right	**Left**	**Normal**
Flexion	_____	_____	_____
Extension	_____	_____	_____

End-feels

PROM should include an assessment of end-feels. Provide a force at the end of the PROM and note the sensation. Record the physiological end-feel for the movement indicated, and note whether a pathological end-feel is present.

	Physiological End-feel	**Pathological End-feel (If Present)**
Flexion	_____	_____
Extension	_____	_____

Resisted Range of Motion

Complete resisted range of motion (RROM) for the movements listed here. Position your patient as indicated, and stabilize the joint to prevent unwanted movement.

Resistive movements should include concentric, eccentric, and isometric muscle actions. Identify prime movers as you complete the assessment.

Range of Motion and Position	Movements (Concentric, Eccentric, and Isometric)	Prime Movers
Knee flexion—lying prone	_____	_____
Knee extension—short sitting	_____	_____

ACTIVITY 5 Joint Stability Tests

Introduction

Injury to ligaments supporting a joint can be identified through stability tests. During these stability tests, *laxity,* or the amount of movement allowed by a joint's capsule and/or ligaments, is compared bilaterally. In addition, the *end-feel,* or sensation felt by the examiner at the limit of the stability test, is noted. Generally speaking, the end-feel during a stability test of a healthy joint is firm and definite, whereas the end-feel of an injured joint is soft and indefinite.

Instructions ➤ Provide the name for the stability test designed to test the given ligament, and then perform each test using classmates as patients. If more than one blank is included, provide alternative tests. Inherent variability of laxity exists among the healthy population. Complete the stability tests on several subjects until you have identified classmates with different grades of laxity. When two classmates with differences in laxity have been identified, you can perform the stability tests to get a better feel for a positive sign of laxity. In an actual injury assessment, this comparison would be made bilaterally.

After completing the assignment, discuss with your partner any joint position changes that should be performed before the stability test (e.g., flexion, rotation). Discuss the purpose for these changes in joint position.

Stabilizing Structures	Stability Tests
Anterior cruciate ligament (ACL)	_____
	_____
Posterior cruciate ligament (PCL)	_____
	_____
	_____
	_____
Medial collateral ligament (MCL)	_____
Lateral collateral ligament (LCL)	_____
Proximal tibiofibular syndesmosis	_____

Type of Instability	
Anterolateral rotatory instability (ALRI)	_____
	_____
	_____

ACTIVITY 6   Special Tests

Introduction

Certain specific injuries and conditions, such as iliotibial band friction syndrome, require special tests that do not fit into the other assessment categories. These are often designed to stress a specific structure through scripted movements.

Instructions ➤ Provide the name for or describe (if there is no specific name) the special test or tests that may be used to identify the injuries and conditions listed here. Complete the special tests using your partner as the injured athlete. Describe a positive sign, and record this information in the space provided. If more than one blank is included, provide alternative tests.

Injury/Condition	Special Test	Positive Sign
Torn meniscus	_____	_____
	_____	_____
	_____	_____
Patellar subluxation	_____	_____
Chondromalacia patella	_____	_____
Medial synovial plica syndrome	_____	_____
Joint effusion	_____	_____
	_____	_____
	_____	_____
Patellar tendinitis	_____	_____
Iliotibial band friction syndrome	_____	_____
	_____	_____
Osteochondral defects	_____	_____

ACTIVITY 7   Neurologic Tests

Instructions ➤ Complete a thorough neurologic assessment for the knee by completing the tests outlined in the following chart. Include dermatome, myotome, and reflex testing.

Nerve Root	Dermatome	Sensory Nerve	Myotome	Motor Nerve	Reflex
L2	Proximal/anterior thigh	Femoral	Hip flexion	Lumbar plexus	Partial patellar
L3	Distal/anterior thigh	Femoral	Knee extension	Femoral	Partial patellar
L4	Medial leg, first toe	Saphenous	Dorsiflexion	Deep peroneal	
L5	Anterior leg, second through fourth toes	Peroneal	Toe extension	Deep peroneal	Patellar

Nerve Root	Dermatome	Sensory Nerve	Myotome	Motor Nerve	Reflex
S1	Lateral leg/foot; Achilles	Peroneal	Plantar flexion	Tibial	Achilles
S2	Posterior leg	Femoral cutaneous	None	Lateral plantar	Achilles

ACTIVITY 8   Skill Integration: Knee

Scenario   A gymnast walks into the athletic training room complaining that her knee "gave out again" when she landed "funny" on a dismount. Demonstrate and explain your assessment of this injury. The model will not respond to your questions but will perform any actions that you request.

Optional: You have _____ minutes to complete your evaluation.

Evaluation

Name: _____   *Date:* _____

History

Establishes mechanism of injury	YES	☐	NO	☐
Establishes specific prior history (to either knee)	YES	☐	NO	☐
Establishes location of pain	YES	☐	NO	☐
Establishes type of pain	YES	☐	NO	☐
Asks if "pop" was felt or heard	YES	☐	NO	☐

Inspection

Inspects for the following:

Swelling	YES	☐	NO	☐
Scars	YES	☐	NO	☐
Obvious deformity	YES	☐	NO	☐
Discoloration	YES	☐	NO	☐
Gait abnormalities	YES	☐	NO	☐
States that observation occurs bilaterally	YES	☐	NO	☐

Palpation

Palpates for presence of the following:

Point tenderness	YES	☐	NO	☐
Temperature change	YES	☐	NO	☐
Swelling (ballotable patella, sweep test)	YES	☐	NO	☐
Deformity	YES	☐	NO	☐
Performs all palpation bilaterally (or states would do so)	YES	☐	NO	☐

Palpates bony and ligamentous structures:

Medial joint line	YES	☐	NO	☐
Medial collateral ligament	YES	☐	NO	☐
Medial femoral condyle/epicondyle	YES	☐	NO	☐
Patella	YES	☐	NO	☐
Tibial tuberosity	YES	☐	NO	☐
Fibular head	YES	☐	NO	☐
Lateral collateral ligament	YES	☐	NO	☐
Lateral joint line	YES	☐	NO	☐
Lateral femoral condyle/epicondyle	YES	☐	NO	☐

Palpates other soft tissue:

Pes anserine tendon group	YES	☐	NO	☐
Semitendinosus tendon	YES	☐	NO	☐
Patellar tendon	YES	☐	NO	☐
Iliotibial band	YES	☐	NO	☐

Popliteal fossa ....YES ☐ NO ☐

Hamstring muscles ....YES ☐ NO ☐

Distal quadriceps ....YES ☐ NO ☐

Range-of-Motion Testing

Response is incorrect if all motions (flexion and extension) are not included. Action must be performed correctly (i.e., proper hand placement, adequate resistance, elimination of substituting movements).

Evaluates AROM ....YES ☐ NO ☐

Evaluates PROM ....YES ☐ NO ☐

Evaluates RROM (or states would not do because of acuteness) ....YES ☐ NO ☐

Performs all ROM bilaterally (or states would do so) ....YES ☐ NO ☐

Ligamentous and Capsular Tests

Response is incorrect if test is not performed correctly (i.e., proper hand placement, appropriate direction and amount of stress).

Performs Lachman test ....YES ☐ NO ☐

Performs valgus stress test (full extension) ....YES ☐ NO ☐

Performs valgus stress test (20 to 30 degrees flexion) ....YES ☐ NO ☐

Performs varus stress test (full extension) ....YES ☐ NO ☐

Performs varus stress test (20 to 30 degrees flexion) ....YES ☐ NO ☐

Performs patellar apprehension test (note: covered in Chapter 6) ....YES ☐ NO ☐

Performs anterior drawer test ....YES ☐ NO ☐

Performs posterior drawer or Godfrey test (or both) ....YES ☐ NO ☐

Performs anterior drawer test with tibial internal and external rotation ....YES ☐ NO ☐

Performs lateral pivot shift (or another anterolateral rotatory instability test) ....YES ☐ NO ☐

Performs all tests bilaterally (or states would do so) ....YES ☐ NO ☐

Special Tests

Response is incorrect if test is not performed correctly (i.e., proper hand position, appropriate direction and amount of stress).

Performs McMurray test ....YES ☐ NO ☐

Performs Apley's compression/distraction test ....YES ☐ NO ☐

Presentation

Performs evaluation in a confident, professional manner ....YES ☐ NO ☐

Performs evaluation in a logical sequence ....YES ☐ NO ☐

Performs evaluation within allotted time ....YES ☐ NO ☐

TOTAL: _____ / _____

Evaluator: _____

Comments: _____

ACTIVITY 9 Skill Integration: Patella

Scenario   You are the athletic trainer for a local running club. A member of the club comes to your clinic complaining of anterior knee pain of 2 months' duration. She has a prescription from her physician for you to "evaluate and treat." Demonstrate and explain your assessment of this injury. The model will not respond to your questions but will perform any actions that you request.

Optional: You have _____ minutes to complete your evaluation.

Evaluation

Name: _____ *Date:* _____

History

Obtains description of onset of symptoms	YES ☐	NO ☐
Establishes specific prior history (to either knee)	YES ☐	NO ☐
Establishes location of pain	YES ☐	NO ☐
Establishes type of pain	YES ☐	NO ☐
Establishes training pattern/changes in pattern	YES ☐	NO ☐
Establishes change in shoe wear, age of shoes	YES ☐	NO ☐
Establishes treatment since onset of symptoms	YES ☐	NO ☐
Establishes physician's diagnosis	YES ☐	NO ☐

Inspection

Inspects for the following:

Swelling	YES ☐	NO ☐
Scars	YES ☐	NO ☐
Obvious deformity	YES ☐	NO ☐
Discoloration	YES ☐	NO ☐
Gait abnormalities	YES ☐	NO ☐
Lower extremity alignment (i.e., Q angle)	YES ☐	NO ☐
Shoe wear pattern/calluses	YES ☐	NO ☐
Standing leg length difference	YES ☐	NO ☐
States that observation occurs bilaterally	YES ☐	NO ☐

Palpation

Palpates for presence of the following:

Point tenderness	YES ☐	NO ☐
Temperature change	YES ☐	NO ☐
Swelling	YES ☐	NO ☐
Deformity	YES ☐	NO ☐
Performs all palpation bilaterally (or states would do so)	YES ☐	NO ☐

Palpates bony and ligamentous structures:

Medial joint line	YES ☐	NO ☐
Medial collateral ligament (MCL)	YES ☐	NO ☐
Medial femoral condyle/epicondyle	YES ☐	NO ☐
Patella/accessible facets	YES ☐	NO ☐
Tibial tuberosity	YES ☐	NO ☐
Fibular head	YES ☐	NO ☐
Lateral collateral ligament (LCL)	YES ☐	NO ☐
Lateral joint line	YES ☐	NO ☐

(Continued)

Lateral femoral condyle/epicondyle .... YES ☐   NO ☐

Palpates other soft tissue:

Pes anserine tendons .... YES ☐   NO ☐

Semitendinosus tendon .... YES ☐   NO ☐

Patellar tendon .... YES ☐   NO ☐

Iliotibial band .... YES ☐   NO ☐

Popliteal fossa .... YES ☐   NO ☐

Hamstring muscles .... YES ☐   NO ☐

Distal quadriceps .... YES ☐   NO ☐

Range-of-Motion Testing

Response is incorrect if all motions (flexion and extension) are not included. Action must be performed correctly (i.e., proper hand placement, adequate resistance, elimination of substituting movements).

Evaluates AROM .... YES ☐   NO ☐

Evaluates PROM .... YES ☐   NO ☐

Evaluates RROM .... YES ☐   NO ☐

Performs all ROM bilaterally (or states would do so) .... YES ☐   NO ☐

Ligamentous and Capsular Testing

Response is incorrect if test is not performed correctly (i.e., proper hand placement, appropriate direction and amount of stress).

Performs single-plane knee stress testing .... YES ☐   NO ☐

Performs test for meniscal pathology .... YES ☐   NO ☐

Assesses patellar glide (medial and lateral) .... YES ☐   NO ☐

Assesses patellar tilt .... YES ☐   NO ☐

Performs all tests bilaterally (or states would do so) .... YES ☐   NO ☐

Special Tests

Response is incorrect if test is not performed correctly (i.e., proper hand position, appropriate direction and amount of stress).

Performs patellar apprehension test .... YES ☐   NO ☐

Performs stutter test .... YES ☐   NO ☐

Presentation

Performs evaluation in a confident, professional manner .... YES ☐   NO ☐

Performs evaluation in a logical sequence .... YES ☐   NO ☐

Performs evaluation within allotted time .... YES ☐   NO ☐

TOTAL: _____ / _____

Evaluator: _____

Comments: _____

_____

_____

ACTIVITY 10   Practical Questions

Instructions ➤ After reading the chapters in your textbook dealing with the knee and completing the corresponding activities, complete the following questions using your lab partner as the patient. The performance evaluation sheets that follow can be used by your instructor to grade the quality of your response to each question.

1. Assess medial and lateral stability at the knee. For each test, include the name, description, and positive signs.

2. Assess the integrity of the anterior cruciate ligament with two tests described in the textbook. For each test, include the name, description, and positive signs. Include three tests for anterolateral rotary instability (ALRI).

3. Assess the integrity of the posterior cruciate ligament with three tests described in the textbook. For each test, include the name, description, and positive signs.

4. Assess AROM at the knee. Include normal values, and identify how you can tell if ROM is abnormal. After completing the active movements, assess PROM and identify the physiological end-feel for each anatomical movement.

5. Complete a thorough assessment of RROM at the knee. Include a prime mover for each anatomical movement.

6. Perform and describe the special tests used to evaluate for meniscal tears. Include the name of each test, a description of the test, and the positive signs of cartilage damage.

7. Your patient has sustained a quadriceps contusion. Conduct a specific evaluation that would identify swelling and loss of ROM.

8. Inspect your patient's knee. Identify and describe any anatomical deformities at the knee, including all possible deformities at the knee (whether the patient has them or not) and any possible injury that the patient will be predisposed to with each type of deformity.

9. Perform and describe two tests for joint effusion. Include the name of each test and what will be a positive sign for joint effusion. Indicate injuries that may occur with joint effusion.

10. Your patient is complaining of general patella pain. Perform and describe special tests that could be used to identify the cause of pain. Include the name of each test and what will be a positive sign.

11. Your patient is complaining of general knee pain. Ask five specific questions that would help identify the specific cause of the pain. Provide a specific answer to each question that you may expect, and indicate what that answer might lead you to suspect.

12. Your patient has a genu varum deformity and complains of lateral knee pain as a result of excessive running. What injury do you suspect? Perform and describe all special tests that could help identify this condition. Include the name of each test and what will be a positive sign.

PERFORMANCE EVALUATION SHEETS

1. *Assess medial and lateral stability at the knee. For each test include the name, description, and positive signs.*

Performance evaluation

	Structure	With Rotation	With Flexion	Description
_____ Valgus	_____	_____	_____	_____
	Hand placement _____		Support leg/guarding _____	

	Structure	With Rotation	With Flexion	Description
_____ Varus	_____	_____	_____	_____
	Hand placement _____		Support leg/guarding _____	

POSITIVE SIGN

_____ Pain   _____ Laxity   _____ Soft end-feel

Bilateral comparison _____

2. *Assess the integrity of the anterior cruciate ligament with two tests described in the textbook. For each test include the name, description, and positive signs. Include three tests for anterolateral rotary instability (ALRI).*

Performance evaluation

	Description			
_____ Anterior drawer	_____			
	_____ Stabilize leg	_____ Thumbs on joint line	_____ Relax hamstrings	

	Flexion	Extension	Description
_____ Lachman test	_____	_____	_____

POSITIVE SIGN

_____ Pain   _____ Laxity   _____ Soft end-feel

	Test	Description	Positive Sign
_____ Pivot shift	_____	_____	_____
_____ Slocum drawer test	_____	_____	_____
_____ Crossover test	_____	_____	_____

Bilateral comparison _____

3. *Assess the integrity of the posterior cruciate ligament with three tests described in the textbook. For each test include the name, description, and positive signs.*

   Performance evaluation

Description		
_____ Posterior drawer	_____	
_____ Stabilize leg	_____ Thumbs on joint line	_____ Relax muscles

	With Rotation	Flexion	Extension	Description
_____ Lachman test	_____	_____	_____	_____

POSITIVE SIGN

_____ Pain	_____ Laxity	_____ Soft end-feel

	Test	Description	Positive Sign
_____ Godfrey test	_____	_____	_____

Bilateral comparison _____

4. *Assess AROM at the knee. Include normal values, and identify how you can tell if ROM is abnormal. After completing the active movements, assess PROM and identify the physiological end-feel for each anatomical movement.*

   Performance evaluation

	Normal Values	Goniometer	Fulcrum	Arms
Flexion	(135–145) _____	_____	_____	_____
Extension	(0) _____	_____	_____	_____
Knee flexed for internal and external rotation _____				

Physiological End-feel	
Flexion	_____
Extension	_____

Bilateral comparison _____

5. *Complete a thorough assessment of RROM at the knee. Include a prime mover for each anatomical movement.*

   Performance evaluation

	Test	Prime Mover
Flexion	_____	_____
Extension	_____	_____
Knee flexed for internal and external rotation	_____	
Active _____	Resistive _____	
Isometric/breaking point test _____	Concentric _____	Eccentric _____
Bilateral comparison _____		

6. *Perform and describe the special tests used to evaluate for meniscal tears. Include the name of each test, a description of the test, and the positive signs of cartilage damage.*

Performance evaluation

	Description	Positive Sign	Stabilize Femur
_____ Apley's compression test	_____	_____	
_____ Apley's distraction test	_____	_____	_____

Internal rotation = lateral meniscus and external rotation = medial rotation

or

Location of pain indicates portion of
meniscus involved _____ _____

Bilateral comparison _____

	Description	Test
_____ McMurray test	_____	_____

	Positive Sign	Flexion/ Extension	Internal/ External Rotation	Valgus
	_____	_____	_____	_____

Bilateral comparison _____

7. *Your patient has sustained a quadriceps contusion. Conduct a specific evaluation that would identify swelling and loss of ROM.*

Performance evaluation

	Normal Values	Goniometer	Fulcrum	Arms
Flexion	(135–145) _____	_____	_____	_____
Extension	(0) _____	_____	_____	_____

Bilateral comparison _____

Did not do unnecessary movements _____

	6 Inches above Joint	4 Inches above Joint	(or)	Over Contusion
Girth measurements	_____	_____		_____

Did not do unnecessary measurements _____

Bilateral comparison _____

8. *Inspect your patient's knee. Identify and describe any anatomical deformities at the knee, including all possible deformities at the knee, whether the patient has them or not, and any possible injury that the patient will be predisposed to with each type of deformity.*

Performance evaluation

	Description	Potential injury
_____ Genu valgum (knock-knee)	_____	_____ (Pes anserinus)
_____ Genu varum (bowleg)	_____	_____ (IT band)
_____ Genu recurvatum	_____	_____ (Hyperextension)
_____ Patella alta	_____	
_____ Patella baja	_____	
_____ Squinting patella	_____	
_____ Frog-eyed patella	_____	
Patella deformities may predispose patient to patella tracking problems or chondromalacia patella	_____	_____

9. *Perform and describe two tests for joint effusion. Include the name of each test and what will be a positive sign for joint effusion. Indicate injuries that may occur with joint effusion.*

Performance evaluation

	Test	Description	Positive Sign
_____ Sweep test	_____	_____	_____
_____ Ballotable patella	_____	_____	_____
Bilateral comparison _____			

Injuries	
Meniscus	_____
Capsular ligament sprains	_____
Torn capsule	_____
Plica syndrome	_____
Suprapatellar or infrapatellar bursitis	_____
Articular fracture	_____

10. *Your patient is complaining of general patella pain. Perform and describe special tests that could be used to identify the cause of pain. Include the name of each test and what will be a positive sign.*

Performance evaluation

	Description	Test	Injury	Positive Sign
_____ Apprehension test	_____	_____	_____	_____
_____ Clarke's sign	_____	_____	_____	_____
_____ Palpation/ patellar movement	_____	_____	_____	_____
_____ Plica syndrome test	_____	_____	_____	_____

Bilateral comparison _____

11. *Your patient is complaining of general knee pain. Ask five specific questions that would help identify the specific cause of the pain. Provide a specific answer to each question that you may expect, and indicate what that answer might lead you to suspect.*

Performance evaluation

Questions	Answers	Example
_____ Mechanism of injury	_____	_____
_____ Location of pain	_____	_____
_____ Type of pain	_____	_____
_____ What worsens or relieves pain	_____	_____
_____ Previous injury	_____	_____
_____ Onset of swelling	_____	_____
_____ Locking or giving way	_____	_____
_____ Sound associated with injury	_____	_____
_____ Other	_____	_____

12. *Your patient has a genu varum deformity and complains of lateral knee pain as a result of excessive running. What injury do you suspect? Perform and describe all special tests that could help identify this condition. Include the name of each test and what will be a positive sign.*

Performance evaluation

_____ IT band friction syndrome

	Description	Test	Positive Sign
_____ Noble's compression test	_____	_____	_____
_____ Ober test	_____	_____	_____

Bilateral comparison _____

ANSWER KEY

Activity 4 — End-feels

Flexion	Usually soft, sometimes firm
Extension	Firm

Activity 5

Anterior cruciate ligament (ACL)	Anterior drawer test
	Lachman test
Posterior cruciate ligament (PCL)	Posterior drawer test
	Godfrey test
Medial collateral ligament (MCL)	Valgus stress test
Lateral collateral ligament (LCL)	Varus stress test
Proximal tibiofibular syndesmosis	Tibiofibular translation test
Anterolateral rotatory instability (ALRI)	Slocum drawer test
	Crossover test
	Pivot shift test

Activity 6

Torn meniscus	Apley's compression and distraction test	Pain with compression; pain reduced on distraction
	McMurray test	Pain; popping, clicking, or locking
Patellar subluxation	Apprehension test	Quadriceps contraction and apprehension
Chondromalacia patella	Clarke's sign	Pain during quadriceps contraction
Medial synovial plica syndrome	Medial femoral plica test	Reproduction of symptoms
Joint effusion	Stutter test	Irregular patellar motion between 40 and 60 degrees
	Sweep test	Fluid moves freely from medial to lateral
	Ballotable patella	Patella bounces back to original position
Patellar tendinitis	Resistive knee extension	Pain
Iliotibial band friction syndrome	Noble's compression test	Pain at lateral femoral condyle

	Ober test	Leg does not adduct past 90 degrees
Osteochondral defects	Wilson's sign	Pain at 30 degrees of flexion relieved with external tibial rotation

Chapter 4

Assessing the Hip, Thigh, and Pelvis

CHAPTER OUTLINE

Activity 8 ➤   PRACTICAL QUESTIONS

Instructions

PERFORMANCE EVALUATION SHEETS

ANSWER KEY

Activity 4: End-feels

Activity 5

ACTIVITY 1   History

Instructions ➤   Have your partner select a common acute injury from the body part that you are studying. Ask a series of questions in an attempt to narrow the injury possibilities and guide the assessment. Your partner should provide the answers that would be likely from an athlete who sustained this injury. Record all questions and responses, and discuss your conclusions with your partner and your instructor. Repeat the process using a chronic injury.

Acute Injury

Question: _____

Response: _____

Question: _____

Response: _____

Question: _____

Response: _____

Question: _____

Response: _____

Question: _____

Response: _____

Question: _____

Response: _____

Question: _____

Response: _____

Question: _____

Response: _____

Question: _____

Response: _____

Question: _____

Response: _____

Chronic Injury

Question: _____

Response: _____

Question: _____

Response: _____

Question: _____

Response: _____

Question: _____

Response: _____

Question: _____

Response: _____

Question: _____

Response: _____

Question: _____

Response: _____

Question: _____

Response: _____

Question: _____

Response: _____

Question: _____

Response: _____

Activity 2   Inspection

Instructions ➤   Obtaining quantitative measurements may be necessary to directly identify conditions or to identify predisposing factors important in the overall assessment. Complete the following measurements on your partner, and compare the measurements bilaterally when appropriate. Compare these measurements with those of other classmates and with normal values. If pathological values are found, discuss the implications for orthopedic injury and possible methods of intervention.

Leg Length Discrepancies

Discrepancies in leg length can be due to differences in the length of the bones (femur or tibia) bilaterally, referred to as an anatomical or true difference. To assess anatomical leg length, compare the distance from the medial malleolus to the anterior superior iliac spine (ASIS) bilaterally (Fig. 4–1). To determine which bone is longer, inspect your patient from the side while he or she is in the hook-lying position. If the knee protrudes anteriorly, the femur is longer; if the knee protrudes superiorly, the tibia is longer (Fig. 4–2).

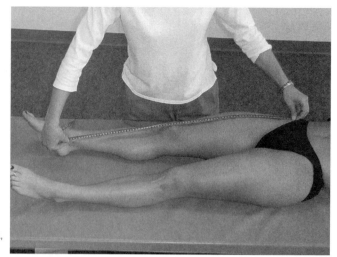

Figure 4–1 Testing for the presence of a true leg length discrepancy. Discrepancies greater than 0.25 inch are considered significant. (From Starkey, C, and Ryan, J: Evaluation of Orthopedic and Athletic Injuries, ed 2. FA Davis, Philadelphia, 2002, with permission.)

Figure 4–2 Clinical discrimination between femoral and tibial leg length differences. *(A)* When viewed from the side, an increased anterior position of one knee indicates a discrepancy in the lengths of the femurs. *(B)* When viewed from the front, a difference in height indicates a discrepancy in the lengths of the tibias. (Adapted from Hoppenfeld, S: Physical examination of the hip and pelvis. In Hoppenfeld, S: Physical Examination of the Spine and Extremities. Appleton-Century Crofts, New York, 1976, p 165, with permission.)

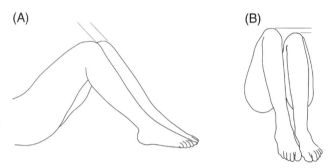

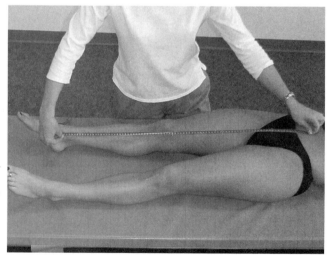

Figure 4–3 Testing for the presence of an apparent leg length discrepancy. This test is meaningful only if the test for true leg length discrepancy is negative. (From Starkey, C, and Ryan, J: Evaluation of Orthopedic and Athletic Injuries, ed 2. FA Davis, Philadelphia, 2002, with permission.)

Apparent discrepancies in leg length, also measurable, are typically caused by pelvic obliquity. These are aptly called functional or apparent discrepancies. To assess functional leg length, compare the distance from the umbilicus to the medial malleolus bilaterally (Fig. 4–3).

Record lengths for the following to identify any leg length discrepancies (in centimeters):

	Discrepancy
PARTNER	
Right ASIS to right malleolus	
Left ASIS to left malleolus	
Umbilicus to right malleolus	
Umbilicus to left malleolus	
CLASSMATE	
Right ASIS to right malleolus	
Left ASIS to left malleolus	
Umbilicus to right malleolus	
Umbilicus to left malleolus	

If you find a classmate who has a true leg length discrepancy, use the measured block to (1) bring the pelvis into horizontal alignment and (2) determine the amount of correction that is needed.

Activity 3   Palpation

Bony Palpation

Instructions ➤ Review the sections on bony anatomy in your textbook before completing this exercise. Begin by locating each bony landmark listed on Fig. 4–4, using the help of your textbook when needed. Develop a systematic approach so that no important structures are missed. Complete the remainder of the assignment after taking a break.

Without the aid of your textbook or skeleton, locate each bony landmark on your partner. When you have found the landmark, mark its location with a small sticker and place a check next to the landmark listed here. Use available resources (e.g., textbook, skeleton, instructor) to check the accuracy of your palpation.

☐ ASIS
☐ Posterior superior iliac spine (PSIS)
☐ Iliac crest
☐ Ischial tuberosity
☐ Greater trochanter

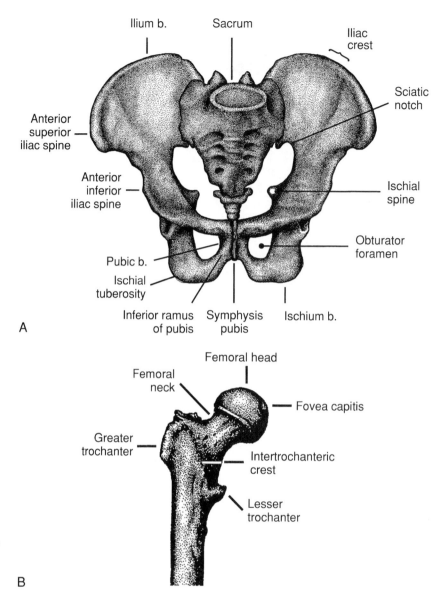

Figure 4–4 *(A)* Pelvis, anterior view. *(B)* Femoral head and neck. (From Starkey, C, and Ryan, J: Evaluation of Orthopedic and Athletic Injuries, ed 2. FA Davis, Philadelphia, 2002, with permission.)

Soft Tissue Palpation

Instructions ➤ Review the sections on soft tissue anatomy of the knee in your textbook before completing this exercise. Begin by locating each structure in a figure in your textbook. Develop a systematic approach so that no important structures are missed. Complete the remainder of the assignment after taking a break.

Without the aid of your textbook or skeleton, locate each structure on your partner. When you have found the landmark, mark its location with a small sticker and place a check next to the landmark listed here. For lengthy or larger structures, mark a prominent portion. Use available resources (e.g., textbook, skeleton, instructor) to check the accuracy of your palpation markers.

☐ Adductor muscle group
☐ Sartorius

☐ Rectus femoris
☐ Gluteus medius
☐ Tensor fasciae latae
☐ Gluteus maximus
☐ Hamstring muscles
☐ Sciatic nerve
☐ Femoral triangle

ACTIVITY 4   Range-of-Motion Tests

Instructions ➤   Ask your patient to complete active range of motion (AROM) for the movements listed here. Note the available range of motion (ROM) and any discomfort.

Passive Range of Motion

After assessing AROM, assess passive range of motion (PROM) for the movements listed here. Compare the results bilaterally and with the normal ROMs reported in your textbook.

	Range of Motion (Degrees)		
	Right	**Left**	**Normal**
HIP			
Flexion			
Extension			
Abduction			
Adduction			
Internal rotation			
External rotation			

End-feels

PROM should include an assessment of end-feels. Provide a force at the end of the PROM and note the sensation. Record the physiological end-feel for the movement indicated, and note whether a pathological end-feel is present.

	Physiological End-feel	Pathological End-feel (If Present)
Flexion		
Extension		
Abduction		
Adduction		
Internal rotation		
External rotation		

Resisted Range of Motion

Complete resisted range of motion (RROM) for the movements listed here. Position your patient as indicated, and stabilize the joint to prevent unwanted movement. Resistive movements should include concentric, eccentric, and isometric muscle actions. Identify prime movers as you complete the assessment.

Range of Motion and Position	Movements (Concentric, Eccentric, and Isometric)	Prime Movers
HIP		
Flexion–short sitting	_____	_____
Extension–lying prone	_____	_____
Abduction–side-lying	_____	_____
Adduction–side-lying with opposite leg held in abduction	_____	_____
Internal rotation–short sitting	_____	_____
External rotation–short sitting	_____	_____

ACTIVITY 5   Special Tests

Introduction

Certain specific injuries and conditions, such as those affecting the hip flexors, require special tests that do not fit into the other assessment categories. These tests are often designed to stress a specific structure through scripted movements.

Instructions ➤ Provide the name for or describe (if there is no specific name) the special test or tests that may be used to identify the injuries and conditions listed here. Complete the special tests using your partner as the injured athlete. Describe a positive sign, and record this information in the space provided. If more than one blank is included, provide alternative tests.

Injury/Condition	Special Test	Positive Sign
Hip flexor tightness	_____	_____
	_____	_____
Sacroiliac pathology	_____	_____
	_____	_____
	_____	_____
Piriformis syndrome	_____	_____
Osteochondral defects	_____	_____

ACTIVITY 6   Neurologic Tests

Instructions ➤   Complete a thorough neurologic assessment for the pelvis, hip, and thigh by completing the tests outlined in the following chart. Include dermatome, myotome, and reflex testing.

Nerve Root	Dermatome	Sensory Nerve	Myotome	Motor Nerve	Reflex
L1	Anterior; lateral pelvis		Hip flexion	Lumbar plexus	None
L2	Proximal; anterior thigh	Femoral	Hip flexion	Lumbar plexus	Partial patellar
L3	Distal; anterior thigh	Femoral	Knee extension	Femoral	Partial patellar
L4	Medial leg; first toe	Saphenous	Dorsiflexion	Deep peroneal	Patellar
L5	Anterior leg; second through fourth toes	Peroneal	Toe extension	Deep peroneal	Patellar
S1	Lateral leg/foot; Achilles	Peroneal	Plantar flexion	Tibial	Achilles

ACTIVITY 7   Skill Integration: Pelvis and Thigh

Scenario   A 36-year-old female runner comes to your clinic complaining of progressively worsening pain in the buttocks and low back. She is 3 months postpartum. Demonstrate and explain your assessment of this injury. The model will not respond to your questions but will perform any actions that you request.

Optional: You have _____ minutes to complete your evaluation.

Evaluation

Name: _____ *Date:* _____

History		
Establishes any specific mechanism of injury	YES ☐	NO ☐
Establishes duration of pain	YES ☐	NO ☐
Establishes location of pain	YES ☐	NO ☐
Establishes type of pain	YES ☐	NO ☐
Establishes pattern of pain (e.g., during or after workouts, in morning)	YES ☐	NO ☐
Establishes presence/absence of previous injury	YES ☐	NO ☐
Establishes training pattern (or changes in same)	YES ☐	NO ☐
Establishes age/type of exercise shoe	YES ☐	NO ☐

Inspection		
Inspects for the following:		
Swelling (bilateral comparison)	YES ☐	NO ☐
Gait abnormalities	YES ☐	NO ☐
Equal height of anterior superior iliac spine (ASIS) and posterior superior iliac spine (PSIS)	YES ☐	NO ☐
Shoe wear pattern	YES ☐	NO ☐
Atrophy (gluts)	YES ☐	NO ☐
General posture (lower extremity alignment)	YES ☐	NO ☐

Palpation		
Palpates for presence of the following:		
Point tenderness	YES ☐	NO ☐
Swelling	YES ☐	NO ☐
Atrophy	YES ☐	NO ☐
Performs all palpation bilaterally (or states would do so)	YES ☐	NO ☐
Palpates bony and ligamentous structures:		
ASIS	YES ☐	NO ☐
Anterior inferior iliac spine	YES ☐	NO ☐
Iliac crest	YES ☐	NO ☐
Greater trochanter	YES ☐	NO ☐
PSIS	YES ☐	NO ☐
Ischial tuberosity	YES ☐	NO ☐
Sacroiliac joints	YES ☐	NO ☐
Sacrum	YES ☐	NO ☐
Palpates other soft tissue:		
Gluteus medius	YES ☐	NO ☐
Gluteus maximus	YES ☐	NO ☐

Hamstrings	YES	☐	NO	☐
Lumbar paravertebrals	YES	☐	NO	☐

Range-of-Motion Testing

Response is incorrect if all motions (hip flexion/extension, hip abduction/adduction, hip internal/external rotation, lumbar flexion/extension*) are not included. Action must be performed correctly (i.e., proper hand placement, adequate resistance, elimination of substituting movements).

Evaluates AROM	YES	☐	NO	☐
Evaluates PROM	YES	☐	NO	☐
Evaluates RROM	YES	☐	NO	☐
Performs all tests bilaterally (or states would do so)	YES	☐	NO	☐

Special Tests

Response is incorrect if test is performed incorrectly (i.e., proper hand position, appropriate direction and amount of stress).

Ober test	YES	☐	NO	☐
Thomas test (hip flexor tightness)	YES	☐	NO	☐
Lasegue test (SLR)*	YES	☐	NO	☐
Gaenslen test	YES	☐	NO	☐
Sacroiliac compression/distraction test	YES	☐	NO	☐
Faber (or Patrick's) test	YES	☐	NO	☐
Hip scouring	YES	☐	NO	☐
Long sit test	YES	☐	NO	☐
Leg length discrepancy	YES	☐	NO	☐
Performs all tests bilaterally (or states would do so)	YES	☐	NO	☐

Neurologic Assessment

Motor:

L1 (hip flexion)	YES	☐	NO	☐
L2, L3, L4 (knee extension)	YES	☐	NO	☐
L4 (ankle dorsiflexion)	YES	☐	NO	☐
L5 (knee flexion [semimembranosus, semitendinosus], great toe extensor)	YES	☐	NO	☐
S1 (knee flexion [biceps femoris])	YES	☐	NO	☐

Sensory:

L1 (lateral hip, anterior thigh)	YES	☐	NO	☐
L2 (anterior thigh)	YES	☐	NO	☐
L3 (anterior thigh)	YES	☐	NO	☐
L4 (medial lower leg)	YES	☐	NO	☐
L5 (dorsal foot)	YES	☐	NO	☐
S1 (lateral foot)	YES	☐	NO	☐

*Note to evaluator: Students may not have been exposed to low-back evaluation before this assessment.

(Continued)

Reflex:

L2, L3, L4 (patellar tendon) ....YES ☐   NO ☐

L5, S1 (Achilles tendon) ....YES ☐   NO ☐

Presentation				

Performs evaluation in confident, professional manner ....YES ☐   NO ☐

Performs evaluation in logical sequence ....YES ☐   NO ☐

Performs evaluation within allotted time ....YES ☐   NO ☐

TOTAL: _____ / _____

Evaluator: _____

Comments: _____

_____

_____

ACTIVITY 8   Practical Questions

Instructions ➤   After reading the chapters in your textbook dealing with the hip, thigh, and pelvis and completing the corresponding activities, complete the following questions using your lab partner as the patient. The performance evaluation sheets can be used by your instructor to grade the quality of your response to each question.

1. Several deformities that can predispose a patient to injury occur in the area of the hip, thigh, and pelvis. Provide the name and a description and then demonstrate how to measure each deformity.

2. Assess AROM at the hip, thigh, and pelvis. Include normal values, and identify how you can tell if ROM is abnormal. After completing the active movements, assess PROM and identify the physiological end-feel for each anatomical movement.

3. Contractures within the hip flexors can predispose a patient to injury. Identify two injuries that may result from hip contractures, and conduct any special tests that can identify contractures. For each test, include the name, description, and positive sign.

4. Complete a thorough assessment of RROM at the hip, thigh, and pelvis. Include a prime mover for each anatomical movement.

5. Conduct a thorough assessment for sacroiliac dysfunction by completing three tests included in your textbook. For each test, include the name, description, and positive sign.

PERFORMANCE EVALUATION SHEETS

1. *Several deformities that can predispose a patient to injury occur in the area of the hip, thigh, and pelvis. Provide the name and a description and then demonstrate how to measure each deformity.*

Performance evaluation

		Common Name	Pathological Value	Description	Measurement
_____	Anteversion	(Toe in) _____	_____	_____	
_____	Retroversion	(Toe out) _____	_____	_____	
_____	Excessive Q angle		_____	_____	_____
_____	Anatomical leg length discrepancy	(True) _____	_____	_____	_____
_____	Identified whether difference was in tibia or femur				
_____	Apparent leg length discrepancy	(Functional) _____	_____	_____	
_____	Genu varum	(Bowleg) _____			
_____	Genu valgum	(Knock-knee) _____	_____	_____	

Bilateral comparison

2. *Assess AROM at the hip, thigh, and pelvis. Include normal values, and identify how you can tell if ROM is abnormal. After completing the active movements, assess PROM and identify the physiological end-feel for each anatomical movement.*

Performance evaluation

	Normal Values	Goniometer	Fulcrum	Arms
Flexion	(120–130)	_____	_____	_____
Extension	(20–30)	_____	_____	_____
Internal rotation	(35–45)	_____	_____	_____
External rotation	(40–50)	_____	_____	_____
Abduction	(45)	_____	_____	_____
Adduction	(20–30)	_____	_____	_____

Physiological End-Feel	
Flexion	_____
Extension	_____
Internal rotation	_____
External rotation	_____
Abduction	_____
Adduction	_____
Bilateral comparison	_____

(Continued)

3. *Contractures within the hip flexors can predispose a patient to injury. Identify two injuries that may result from hip contractures, and conduct any special tests that can identify contractures. For each test, include the name, description, and positive sign.*

   Performance evaluation

   _____ Hip flexor strains

   _____ Low back injury

   _____ Hip flexor tendinitis

   _____ Iliopsoas bursitis

	Test	Description	Positive Rectus Femoris	Positive Iliopsoas
_____ Kendall test	_____	_____	_____	_____

	Test	Description	Positive Leg Raise	Lordotic Curve
_____ Thomas test	_____	_____	_____	_____

   Bilateral comparison _____

4. *Complete a thorough assessment of RROM at the hip, thigh, and pelvis. Include a prime mover for each anatomical movement.*

   Performance evaluation

	Test	Prime Mover
Flexion	_____	_____
Extension	_____	_____
Internal rotation	_____	_____
External rotation	_____	_____

   Knee flexed for internal and external rotation _____

   Active _____ Resistive _____

   Isometric/breaking point test _____ Concentric _____ Eccentric _____

   Bilateral comparison _____

5. *Conduct a thorough assessment for sacroiliac dysfunction by completing three tests included in your textbook. For each test, include the name, description, and positive sign.*

   Performance evaluation

	Description	Test	Positive Sign
_____ Sacroiliac compression/distraction tests	_____	_____	_____
_____ Patrick's test (Fabere sign)	_____	_____	_____
_____ Gaenslen test	_____	_____	_____

   Bilateral comparison _____

ANSWER KEY

Activity 4

End-feels

Flexion	Usually soft, sometimes firm
Extension	Firm
Abduction	Firm
Adduction	Firm
Internal rotation	Firm
External rotation	Firm

Activity 5

Hip flexor tightness	Thomas test	Rectus femoris—inability to flex knee
	Iliopsoas—leg raises off table	
Sacroiliac (SI) pathology	SI compression and distraction test	SI pain
	Patrick's test	SI pain (fabere sign)
	Gaenslen test	SI pain
Piriformis syndrome	Piriformis syndrome test	Radiating pain
Osteochondral defects	Hip scouring	Pain in hip

Chapter 5

Assessing Posture and Gait

ACTIVITY 1   Posture Assessment

Introduction

This activity will involve a comprehensive assessment of posture for both the lower and upper extremities. Proper documentation of posture is emphasized.

Instructions ➤   Review the guidelines for documenting posture that are presented in your textbook. Using these guidelines and the Standard Postural Assessment Form that follows, complete a thorough postural assessment of your subject. Repeat the process using another classmate of a dissimilar body type.

Standard Postural Assessment Form

Name: _____

Clinician: _____

Painful area: _____

Date: _____

Duration of symptoms (months): _____ **Subject 1**

ANTERIOR VIEW

Alignment of plumb line with trunk: _____

Alignment of plumb line with head: _____

Calluses, bunions, blisters on feet: _____

Lower Extremity

Arch Position:	□ pes planus	□ pes cavus	□ neutral
Subtalar Joint:	□ pronated	□ supinated	□ neutral
Tibia Position:	□ medial rotation	□ lateral rotation	□ neutral
Patella Position	□ squinting	□ frog-eyed	□ neutral
Leg Position:	□ genu valgum	□ genu varum	□ neutral

Q angle: □ left: _____ □ right: _____

Muscle mass/girth comments: _____

Other comments: _____

Pelvis/Trunk

Iliac crest symmetry: _____

ASIS symmetry: _____

Abdominal muscle mass: _____

Chest Shape: □ pectus excavatum □ pectus recurvatum □ normal

Shoulder Girdle, Cervical Spine, and Head

Shoulder Position:	□ internally rotated	□ externally rotated	□ neutral
Shoulder Heights:	□ right elevated right	□ depressed	□ neutral
Head Position:	□ side bent	□ rotated	□ neutral

Pectoral muscle mass: _____

Upper trapezius muscle mass: _____

POSTERIOR VIEW

Alignment of plumb line with trunk: _____

Alignment of plumb line with head: _____

Note calluses, blisters on heels: _____

Lower Extremity

Calcaneal Position:	□ genu valgum	□ genu varum	□ neutral
Leg Position:	□ genu valgum	□ genu varum	□ neutral

Muscle mass calves: _____

Muscle mass posterior thighs: _____

Pelvis/Trunk

Spinal Alignment: □ scoliosis □ neutral

Iliac crest symmetry: _____

PSIS symmetry: _____

Gluteal muscle mass: _____

Shoulder Girdle, Cervical Spine, and Head

Scapula Positions: _____

Elevation/depression: _____

Protraction/retraction: _____

Upward/downward Rotation: _____

Winging: _____

Periscapula muscle mass: _____

Upper trapezius muscle mass: _____

Shoulder height: _____

Head Position: □ side bent □ rotated □ neutral

LATERAL VIEW: RIGHT or LEFT (circle which):

Note Alignment of following structures relative to plumb line:

Lat. Malleolus:	□ anterior	□ posterior	□ bisecting
Talocrural Joint:	□ plantarflexed	□ dorsiflexed	□ neutral
Lat. Femoral Epicondyle:	□ anterior	□ posterior	□ bisecting
Knee Position:	□ flexed	□ extended	□ neutral
Greater Trochanter:	□ anterior	□ posterior	□ bisecting
Mid-Thorax:	□ anterior	□ posterior	□ bisecting
Acromion Process:	□ anterior	□ posterior	□ bisecting
Cervical Vertebral Bodies:	□ anterior	□ posterior	□ bisecting
External Auditory Meatus:	□ anterior	□ posterior	□ bisecting
Pelvic Position:	□ ant. rotation	□ post. rotation	□ neutral
Shoulder Position:	□ forward	□ neutral	
Head Position:	□ forward	□ neutral	

Lumbar Spine Position: _____

Thoracic Spine Position: _____

Cervical Spine Position: _____

Shoulder/Head: _____

LATERAL VIEW: RIGHT or LEFT (circle which):

Note Alignment of following structures relative to plumb line:

Lat. Malleolus:	□ anterior	□ posterior	□ bisecting
Talocrural Joint:	□ plantarflexed	□ dorsiflexed	□ neutral
Lat. Femoral Epicondyle:	□ anterior	□ posterior	□ bisecting
Knee Position:	□ flexed	□ extended	□ neutral
Greater Trochanter:	□ anterior	□ posterior	□ bisecting
Midthorax:	□ anterior	□ posterior	□ bisecting
Acromion Process:	□ anterior	□ posterior	□ bisecting
Cervical Vertebral Bodies:	□ anterior	□ posterior	□ bisecting
External Auditory Meatus:	□ anterior	□ posterior	□ bisecting
Pelvic Position:	□ ant. rotation	□ post. rotation	□ neutral
Shoulder Position:	□ forward	□ neutral	
Head Position:	□ forward	□ neutral	

Lumbar Spine Position: _____

Thoracic Spine Position: _____

Cervical Spine Position: _____

Shoulder/Head: _____

(From Starkey, C, and Ryan, J: Evaluation of Orthopedic and Athletic Injuries, ed 2. FA Davis, Philadelphia, 2002, with permission.)

Standard Postural Assessment Form

Subject 2

Name: _____

Clinician: _____

ANTERIOR VIEW

Alignment of plumb line with trunk: _____

Alignment of plumb line with head: _____

Calluses, bunions, blisters on feet: _____

Lower Extremity

Arch Position:	☐ pes planus	☐ pes cavus	☐ neutral
Subtalar Joint:	☐ pronated	☐ supinated	☐ neutral
Tibia Position:	☐ medial rotation	☐ lateral rotation	☐ neutral
Patella Position	☐ squinting	☐ frog-eyed	☐ neutral
Leg Position:	☐ genu valgum	☐ genu varum	☐ neutral

Q angle: ☐ left: ☐ right:

Muscle mass/girth comments: _____

Other comments: _____

Pelvis/Trunk

Iliac crest symmetry: _____

ASIS symmetry: _____

Abdominal muscle mass: _____

Chest Shape: ☐ pectus excavatum ☐ pectus recurvatum ☐ normal

Shoulder Girdle, Cervical Spine, and Head

Shoulder Position: ☐ internally rotated	☐ externally rotated	☐ neutral
Shoulder Heights: ☐ right elevated right	☐ depressed	☐ neutral
Head Position: ☐ side bent	☐ rotated	☐ neutral

Pectoral muscle mass: _____

Upper trapezius muscle mass: _____

Painful area: _____

Date: _____

POSTERIOR VIEW

Alignment of plumb line with trunk: _____

Alignment of plumb line with head: _____

Note calluses, blisters on heels: _____

Lower Extremity

Calcaneal Position:	☐ genu valgum	☐ genu varum	☐ neutral
Leg Position:	☐ genu valgum	☐ genu varum	☐ neutral

Muscle mass calves: _____

Muscle mass posterior thighs: _____

Pelvis/Trunk

Spinal Alignment: ☐ scoliosis ☐ neutral

Iliac crest symmetry: _____

PSIS symmetry: _____

Gluteal muscle mass: _____

Shoulder Girdle, Cervical Spine, and Head

Scapula Positions: _____

Elevation/depression: _____

Protraction/retraction: _____

Upward/downward Rotation: _____

Winging: _____

Periscapula muscle mass: _____

Upper trapezius muscle mass: _____

Shoulder height: _____

Head Position: ☐ side bent ☐ rotated ☐ neutral

Duration of symptoms (months): _____

LATERAL VIEW: RIGHT or LEFT (circle which):

Note Alignment of following structures relative to plumb line:

Lat. Malleolus:	☐ anterior	☐ posterior	☐ bisecting
Talocrural Joint:	☐ plantarflexed	☐ dorsiflexed	☐ neutral
Lat. Femoral Epicondyle:	☐ anterior	☐ posterior	☐ bisecting
Knee Position:	☐ flexed	☐ extended	☐ neutral
Greater Trochanter:	☐ anterior	☐ posterior	☐ bisecting
Mid-Thorax:	☐ anterior	☐ posterior	☐ bisecting
Acromion Process:	☐ anterior	☐ posterior	☐ bisecting
Cervical Vertebral Bodies:	☐ anterior	☐ posterior	☐ bisecting
External Auditory Meatus:	☐ ant. rotation	☐ post. rotation	☐ bisecting
Pelvic Position:	☐ forward	☐ neutral	
Shoulder Position:	☐ forward	☐ neutral	
Head Position:			

Lumbar Spine Position: _____

Thoracic Spine Position: _____

Cervical Spine Position: _____

Shoulder/Head: _____

LATERAL VIEW: RIGHT or LEFT (circle which):

Note Alignment of following structures relative to plumb line

Lat. Malleolus:	☐ anterior	☐ posterior	☐ bisecting
Talocrural Joint:	☐ plantarflexed	☐ dorsiflexed	☐ neutral
Lat. Femoral Epicondyle:	☐ anterior	☐ posterior	☐ bisecting
Knee Position:	☐ flexed	☐ extended	☐ neutral
Greater Trochanter:	☐ anterior	☐ posterior	☐ bisecting
Midthorax:	☐ anterior	☐ posterior	☐ bisecting
Acromion Process:	☐ anterior	☐ posterior	☐ bisecting
Cervical Vertebral Bodies:	☐ anterior	☐ posterior	☐ bisecting
External Auditory Meatus:	☐ anterior	☐ posterior	☐ bisecting
Pelvic Position:	☐ ant. rotation	☐ post. rotation	☐ neutral
Shoulder Position:	☐ forward	☐ neutral	
Head Position:	☐ forward	☐ neutral	

Lumbar Spine Position: _____

Thoracic Spine Position: _____

Cervical Spine Position: _____

Shoulder/Head: _____

(From Starkey, C, and Ryan, J: Evaluation of Orthopedic and Athletic Injuries, ed 2. FA Davis, Philadelphia, 2002, with permission.)

ACTIVITY 2   Gait Assessment

Introduction

To review the gait cycle, identify the event that marks the beginning and end of each phase in the following table. The event marking the end of one phase will represent the beginning of the subsequent phase.

	Begins With	Ends With
STANCE PHASE		
Initial contact	_____	_____
Loading response	_____	_____
Midstance	_____	_____
Terminal stance	_____	_____
Preswing	_____	_____
SWING PHASE		
Initial swing	_____	_____
Midswing	_____	_____
Terminal swing	_____	_____

Instructions ➤ Before completing this activity, review the guidelines for observational gait analysis presented in your textbook. Observe your patient's walking gait, and record the gross position of each joint during each phase. Note the relative position of each joint from phase to phase. When you have completed the assignment, compare these positions with the norms presented in your textbook. Keep in mind that the precise positions included in your textbook were determined using video analysis.

Phase	Joint	Positions
Initial contact	Subtalar	_____
	Talocrural	_____
	Knee	_____
	Hip	_____
Loading response	Subtalar	_____
	Talocrural	_____
	Knee	_____
	Hip	_____
Midstance	Subtalar	_____
	Talocrural	_____
	Knee	_____
	Hip	_____

Phase	Joint	Positions
Terminal stance	Subtalar	_____
	Talocrural	_____
	Knee	_____
	Hip	_____
Preswing	Subtalar	_____
	Talocrural	_____
	Knee	_____
	Hip	_____
Initial swing	Subtalar	_____
	Talocrural	_____
	Knee	_____
	Hip	_____
Midswing	Subtalar	_____
	Talocrural	_____
	Knee	_____
	Hip	_____
Terminal swing	Subtalar	_____
	Talocrural	_____
	Knee	_____
	Hip	_____

ACTIVITY 3   Practical Questions

Instructions ➤   After reading the chapters in your textbook dealing with posture and gait and completing the corresponding activities, complete the following questions using your lab partner as the patient. The performance evaluation sheets can be used by your instructor to grade the quality of your response to each question.

1. Take several walking strides in slow motion. Describe the five parts of the stance phase and three parts of the swing phase by pausing at the appropriate point and naming the subphase.

2. Freeze during one of the eight subphases and describe the position of the subtalar, talocrural, knee, and hip joints.

PERFORMANCE EVALUATION SHEETS

1. *Take several walking strides in slow motion. Describe the five parts of the stance phase and three parts of the swing phase by pausing at the appropriate point and naming the subphase.*

Performance evaluation

STANCE PHASE

Initial contact _____

Loading response _____

Midstance _____

Terminal stance _____

Preswing _____

SWING PHASE

Initial swing _____

Midswing _____

Terminal swing _____

2. *Freeze during one of the eight subphases and describe the position of the subtalar, talocrural, knee, and hip joints.*

Performance evaluation

Chosen Subphase	Joint	Anatomical Position
_____	Subtalar	_____
	Talocrural	_____
	Knee	_____
	Hip	_____

Assessing the Spine

Activity 7 ➤ PRACTICAL QUESTIONS

Instructions

PERFORMANCE EVALUATION SHEETS

ANSWER KEY

Activity 5

ACTIVITY 1 History

Instructions ➤ Have your partner select a common acute injury from the body part that you are studying. Ask a series of questions in an attempt to narrow the injury possibilities and guide the assessment. Your partner should provide the answers that would be likely from an athlete who sustained this injury. Record all questions and responses, and discuss your conclusions with your partner and your instructor. Questions concerning pain should address the following, which are presented with the easy-to-remember O, P, Q, R, S, T system. Repeat the process using a chronic injury.

Onset—rapid or gradual
Provocative—what improves or worsens
Quality—type
Radiation
Site—where
Timing—when

Acute Injury

Question: _____
Response: _____

Question: _____
Response: _____

Question: _____
Response: _____

Question: _____
Response: _____

Question: _____
Response: _____

Question: _____
Response: _____

Question: _____
Response: _____

Question: _____
Response: _____

Question: _____

Response: _____

Question: _____

Response: _____

Chronic Injury

Question: _____

Response: _____

Question: _____

Response: _____

Question: _____

Response: _____

Question: _____

Response: _____

Question: _____

Response: _____

Question: _____

Response: _____

Question: _____

Response: _____

Question: _____

Response: _____

Question: _____

Response: _____

Question: _____

Response: _____

ACTIVITY 2 Inspection

Instructions ➤ Inspect your patient from an anterior, a posterior, and a lateral direction to assess alignment and curvature.

Alignment

Assess alignment by noting the level of the landmarks that are listed here. Make note of any lack of symmetry, and discuss any implications of such poor alignment with your partner.

☐ Head
☐ Shoulders
☐ Posterior superior iliac spine (PSIS)

☐ Gluteal folds
☐ Popliteal crease
☐ Anterior superior iliac spine (ASIS)

Curvature

Assess the frontal and sagittal curvature of the spine.

There should be no frontal curvature. Any curvature in the frontal plane is scoliosis. To check your patient for structural scoliosis, mark each spinous process and inspect posteriorly. To check for functional scoliosis, have your patient flex the spine slowly while you inspect the line of marked spinous processes.

The spine is curved in the sagittal plane to provide shock absorption. Any deviation from normal for any of these curves may produce stress on the spine, leading to pain and chronic injury. Observe your patient from the side, and note the following curves:

☐ Cervical lordotic curve
☐ Thoracic kyphotic curve
☐ Lumbar lordotic curve

ACTIVITY 3   Palpation

Bony Palpation

Instructions ➤ Review the sections on bony anatomy in your textbook before completing this exercise. Figure 6–1 shows a comparison of cervical, thoracic, and lumbar vertebrae. Develop a systematic approach so that no important structures are missed. Complete the remainder of the assignment after taking a break.

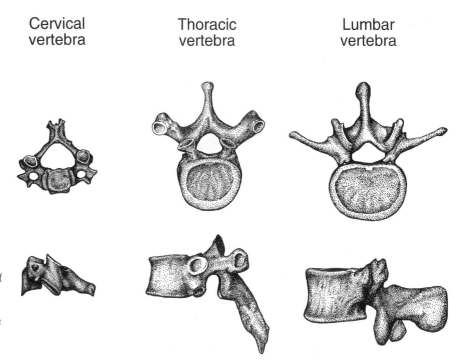

Cervical vertebra   Thoracic vertebra   Lumbar vertebra

Figure 6–1 Comparative anatomy of the cervical, thoracic, and lumbar spines. (From Starkey, C, and Ryan, J: Evaluation of Orthopedic and Athletic Injuries, ed 2. FA Davis, Philadelphia, 2002, with permission.)

Without the aid of your textbook or skeleton, locate each bony landmark on your partner. When you have found the landmark, mark its location with a small sticker and place a check next to the landmark listed here. Use available resources (e.g., textbook, skeleton, instructor) to check the accuracy of your palpation.

☐ Hyoid bone
☐ Occipital bone
☐ Spinous processes
☐ Transverse process

Figure 6–2 illustrates the surface landmarks (with corresponding vertebrae) to assist you with palpation of the vertebrae.

Without the aid of your textbook or skeleton, locate each bony landmark on your partner. When you have found the landmark, mark its location with a small sticker and place a check next to the landmark listed here. Use available resources (e.g., textbook, skeleton, instructor) to check the accuracy of your palpation.

☐ C7 (T1)—vertebra prominens
☐ T2—top of scapula
☐ T4—base of spine of scapula
☐ T7—inferior angle of scapula

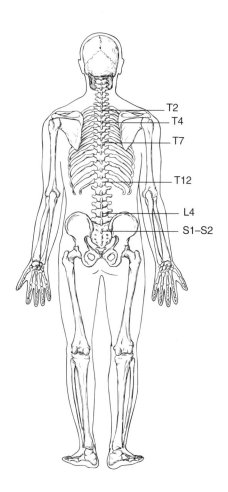

Figure 6–2 Skeleton, posterior view.

☐ T12—lowest rib
☐ L4—top of iliac crest
☐ S1–S2—PSIS

Soft Tissue Palpation

Instructions ➤   Review the sections on soft tissue anatomy of the spine in your textbook before completing this exercise. Begin by locating each structure on a figure in your textbook. Develop a systematic approach so that no important structures are missed. Complete the remainder of the assignment after taking a break.

Without the aid of your textbook or skeleton, locate each structure on your partner. When you have found the landmark, mark its location with a small sticker and place a check next to the landmark listed here. For lengthy or larger structures, mark a prominent portion. Use available resources (e.g., textbook, skeleton, instructor) to check the accuracy of your palpation markers.

Cervical Spine

☐ Thyroid cartilage
☐ Cricoid cartilage
☐ Sternocleidomastoid
☐ Carotid artery
☐ Lymph nodes
☐ Trapezius

Thoracic Spine

☐ Trapezius
☐ Paravertebral muscles

Lumbar Spine

☐ Paravertebral muscles

Sacral Spine

☐ Gluteal muscles
☐ Sciatic nerve

ACTIVITY 4   Range-of-Motion Tests

Instructions ➤   Ask your patient to complete active range of motion (AROM) for the movements listed on page 90. Note the available range of motion (ROM) and any discomfort.

ROM of the spine is the cumulative effect of movement occurring between each pair of adjacent vertebrae. Because there is no single axis of rotation, accurately measuring ROM with a goniometer is difficult. In addition, there is often no means for bilateral comparison. To assess ROM of the spine, simply observe the movement and compare with accepted norms.

Range of Motion	
CERVICAL	
Flexion	_____
Extension	_____
Lateral bending	_____
Rotation	_____
LUMBAR (TRUNK)	
Flexion	_____
Extension	_____
Lateral bending	_____
Rotation	_____

End-feels

Passive range of motion (PROM) should include an assessment of end-feels. Provide a force at the end of the PROM and note the sensation. Record the physiological end-feel for the movement indicated, and note whether a pathological end-feel is present.

	Physiological End-feel	Pathological End-feel (If Present)
CERVICAL		
Flexion	_____	_____
Extension	_____	_____
Lateral bending	_____	_____
Rotation	_____	_____
LUMBAR (TRUNK)		
Flexion	_____	_____
Extension	_____	_____
Lateral bending	_____	_____
Rotation	_____	_____

Resisted Range of Motion

Complete resisted range of motion (RROM) for the movements listed here. Position your patient as indicated, and stabilize the joint to prevent unwanted movement. Resistive movements should include concentric, eccentric, and isometric muscle actions. Identify prime movers as you complete the assessment.

Range of Motion and Position	Movements (Concentric, Eccentric, and Isometric)	Prime Movers
CERVICAL		
Flexion—lying supine		
Extension—lying prone with head extending beyond table		
Lateral bending—short sitting		
Rotation—short sitting		
LUMBAR (TRUNK)		
Flexion—lying supine		
Extension—lying supine		
Lateral bending—side-lying		
Rotation—lying supine		

ACTIVITY 5   Special Tests

Introduction

Certain specific injuries and conditions, such as winging scapula or spondylopathy, require special tests that do not fit into the other assessment categories. These tests are often designed to stress a specific structure through scripted movements.

Instructions ➤ Provide the name for or describe (if there is no specific name) the special test or tests that may be used to identify the injuries and conditions listed here. Complete the special tests using your partner as the injured athlete. Describe a positive sign, and record this information in the space provided. If more than one blank is included, provide alternative tests.

Injury/Condition	Special Test	Positive Sign
CERVICAL		
Cervical nerve root compression		
Upper motor neuron lesions		
Brachial plexus strain		
THORACIC		
Winging scapula		
LUMBAR		
Intervertebral disc lesions		

Injury/Condition	Special Test	Positive Sign
Sciatica	_____	_____
	_____	_____
Spondylopathy	_____	_____

ACTIVITY 6 Neurologic Tests

Instructions ➤ Complete a thorough neurologic assessment for the upper quarter by completing the tests outlined in the following chart. Include dermatome, myotome, and reflex testing.

Nerve Root	Dermatome	Sensory Nerve	Myotome	Motor Nerve	Reflex
C5	Lateral arm	Axillary	Shoulder abduction	Axillary	Biceps
C6	Lateral forearm/ fingers 1 and 2	Musculocu-taneous	Elbow flexion	Musculocu-taneous	Brachioradialis
C7	Third finger	Radial	Elbow extension	Radial	Triceps
C8	Medial forearm/ fingers 4 and 5	Ulnar	Finger flexion	Median/palmar interosseous	None
T1	Medial elbow	Medial brachial cutaneous	None	None	None

Instructions ➤ Complete a thorough neurologic assessment for the lower quarter by completing the tests outlined in the following chart. Include dermatome, myotome, and reflex testing.

Nerve Root	Dermatome	Sensory Nerve	Myotome	Motor Nerve	Reflex
L1	Anterior/lateral pelvis		Hip flexion	Lumbar plexus	None
L2	Proximal/anterior thigh	Femoral	Hip flexion	Lumbar plexus	Partial patellar
L3	Distal/anterior thigh	Femoral	Knee extension	Femoral	Partial patellar
L4	Medial leg/first toe	Saphenous	Dorsiflexion	Deep peroneal	Patellar
L5	Anterior leg/ second through fourth toes	Peroneal	Toe extension	Deep peroneal	Patellar
S1	Lateral leg/foot; Achilles	Peroneal	Plantar flexion	Tibial	Achilles
S2	Posterior leg	Femoral cuta-neous	None	Lateral plantar	Achilles

ACTIVITY 7   Practical Questions

Instructions ➤   After reading the chapters in your textbook dealing with the spine and completing the corresponding activities, complete the following questions using your lab partner as the patient. The performance evaluation sheets can be used by your instructor to grade the quality of your response to each question.

1. Your patient is complaining of general low back pain. Ask six specific questions that will help you identify the specific cause of the pain using the O, P, Q, R, S, T mnemonic.

2. Complete a thorough assessment of RROM at the spine. Include a prime mover for each anatomical movement.

3. Conduct special tests that can be used to identify injury to the sciatic nerve. For each test, include the name, description, and positive signs.

4. Complete a thorough neurologic assessment for the upper quarter. Include the following in your answer: nerve roots being tested, dermatome test and sensory nerve, myotome test and motor nerve, and reflex for each nerve root.

5. Complete a thorough neurologic assessment for the lower quarter. Include the following in your answer: nerve roots being tested, dermatome test and sensory nerve, myotome test and motor nerve, and reflex for each nerve root.

PERFORMANCE EVALUATION SHEETS

1 *Your patient is complaining of general low back pain. Ask six specific questions that would help identify the specific cause of the pain using the O, P, Q, R, S, T mnemonic.*

Performance evaluation

_____ Was the onset of pain rapid or gradual?

_____ What improves or worsens your pain?

_____ What type of pain are you experiencing?

_____ Does your pain radiate?

_____ Where are you experiencing pain?

_____ When do you experience pain?

2. *Complete a thorough assessment of RROM at the spine. Include a prime mover for each anatomical movement.*

Performance evaluation

	Test	Prime Mover
CERVICAL		
Flexion	_____	_____
Extension	_____	_____
Lateral bending	_____	_____
Rotation	_____	_____
LUMBAR (TRUNK)		
Flexion	_____	_____
Extension	_____	_____
Lateral bending	_____	_____
Rotation	_____	_____

3. *Conduct special tests that can be used to identify injury to the sciatic nerve. For each test include the name, description, and positive signs.*

Performance evaluation

	Test	Description	Positive Sign
_____ Lasegue's sign	_____	_____	_____
_____ Bowstring test	_____	_____	_____
_____ Piriformis syndrome test	_____	_____	_____

Etiology of piriformis syndrome _____

Bilateral comparison _____

4. *Complete a thorough neurologic assessment for the upper quarter. Include the following in your answer: nerve roots being tested, dermatome test and sensory nerve, myotome test and motor nerve, and reflex for each nerve root.*

Performance evaluation

Nerve Root	Dermatome	Sensory Nerve	Myotome	Motor Nerve	Reflex
C5	Lateral arm	Axillary	Shoulder abduction	Axillary	Biceps
C6	Lateral forearm/ fingers 1 and 2	Musculocu- taneous	Elbow flexion	Musculocu- taneous	Brachioradialis
C7	Third finger	Radial	Elbow extension	Radial	Triceps
C8	Medial forearm/ fingers 4 and 5	Ulnar	Finger flexion	Median/palmar interosseous	None
T1	Medial elbow	Medial brachial cutaneous	None	None	None

5. *Complete a thorough neurologic assessment for the lower quarter. Include the following in your answer: nerve roots being tested, dermatome test and sensory nerve, myotome test and motor nerve, and reflex for each nerve root.*

Performance evaluation

Nerve Root	Dermatome	Sensory Nerve	Myotome	Motor Nerve	Reflex
L1	Anterior/lateral pelvis		Hip flexion	Lumbar plexus	None
L2	Proximal/anterior thigh	Femoral	Hip flexion	Lumbar plexus	Partial patellar
L3	Distal/anterior thigh	Femoral	Knee extension	Femoral	Partial patellar
L4	Medial leg/first toe	Saphenous	Dorsiflexion	Deep peroneal	Patellar

(Continued)

L5	Anterior leg/second through fourth toes	Peroneal	Toe extension	Deep peroneal	Patellar
S1	Lateral leg/foot; Achilles	Peroneal	Plantar flexion	Tibial	Achilles

ANSWER KEY

Activity 5

CERVICAL

Cervical nerve root compression	Shoulder abduction test	Decreased symptoms
	Cervical compression test	Pain in upper cervical spine
Upper motor neuron lesions	Babinski's test	Great toes extends while others flex
	Oppenheim test	Great toes extends while others flex
Brachial plexus strain	Brachial plexus traction test	Radiating pain opposite stretch

THORACIC

Winging scapula	Wall push-up	Vertebral border of scapula protrudes posteriorly

LUMBAR

Intervertebral disc lesions	Valsalva's test	Spinal or radicular pain
	Wall straight leg raise	Pain opposite leg being raised
	Femoral nerve stretch test	Pain in anterior and lateral thigh
Sciatica	Straight leg raise (Lasegue's)	Radiating pain
	Bowstring test	Radiating pain
Spondylopathy	Single-leg stance test	Lumbar spine or sacroiliac pain

Chapter 7

Assessing the Shoulder

CHAPTER OUTLINE

ACTIVITY 1   History

Instructions ➤   Have your partner select a common acute injury from the body part that you are studying. Ask a series of questions in an attempt to narrow the injury possibilities and guide the assessment. Your partner should provide the answers that would be likely from an athlete who sustained this injury. Record all questions and responses, and discuss your conclusions with your partner and your instructor. Repeat the process using a chronic injury.

Acute Injury

Question: _____

Response: _____

Question: _____

Response: _____

Question: _____

Response: _____

Question: _____

Response: _____

Question: _____

Response: _____

Question: _____

Response: _____

Question: _____

Response: _____

Question: _____

Response: _____

Question: _____

Response: _____

Question: _____

Response: _____

Question: _____

Response: _____

Chronic Injury

Question: _____

Response: _____

Question: _____

Response: _____

Question: _____

Response: _____

Question: _____

Response: _____

Question: _____

Response: _____

Question: _____

Response: _____

Question: _____

Response: _____

Question: _____

Response: _____

Question: _____

Response: _____

Question: _____

Response: _____

ACTIVITY 2 Inspection

Instructions ➤ Define the deformities, abnormalities, and conditions listed here. Inspect your partner's shoulder to identify each condition. Inspect other students until each of the conditions has been found. If a condition is not found within the class population, find a photograph of the deformity in your textbook.

Step deformity _____

Sulcus sign _____

Sprengel's deformity _____

ACTIVITY 3   Palpation

Bony Palpation

Instructions ➤ Review the sections on bony anatomy in your textbook before completing this exercise. Begin by locating each bony landmark listed on Fig. 7–1, using the help of your textbook when needed. Develop a systematic approach so that no important structures are missed. Complete the remainder of the assignment after taking a break.

Without the aid of your textbook or skeleton, locate each bony landmark on your partner. When you have found the landmark, mark its location with a small sticker and place a check next to the landmark listed here. Use available resources (e.g., textbook, skeleton, instructor) to check the accuracy of your palpation.

☐ Sternum
☐ Clavicle
☐ Acromioclavicular (AC) joint
☐ Sternoclavicular (SC) joint
☐ Scapula
   ☐ Acromion process
   ☐ Coracoid process
   ☐ Spine
   ☐ Superior angle
   ☐ Inferior angle
   ☐ Medial border

☐ Humerus
   ☐ Head
   ☐ Greater tuberosity
   ☐ Bicipital groove
   ☐ Lesser tuberosity
   ☐ Shaft

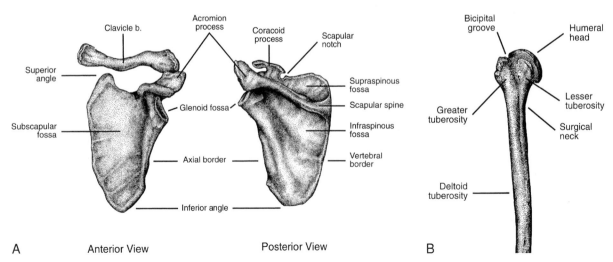

Figure 7–1 Bony anatomy of the shoulder joint. *(A)* Anterior and posterior views of the scapula. *(B)* Upper humerus. (From Starkey, C, and Ryan, J: Evaluation of Orthopedic and Athletic Injuries, ed 2. FA Davis, Philadelphia, 2002, with permission.)

Soft Tissue Palpation

Instructions ➤ Review the sections on soft tissue anatomy of the shoulder in your textbook before completing this exercise. Begin by locating each structure in a figure in your textbook. Develop a systematic approach so that no important structures are missed. Complete the remainder of the assignment after taking a break.

Without the aid of your textbook or skeleton, locate each structure on your partner. When you have found the landmark, mark its location with a small sticker and place a check next to the landmark listed here. For lengthy or large structures, mark a prominent portion. Use available resources (e.g., textbook, skeleton, instructor) to check the accuracy of your palpation markers.

Anterior Muscles

- ☐ Pectoralis major
- ☐ Pectoralis minor
- ☐ Coracobrachialis

Humeral Muscles

- ☐ Deltoids
- ☐ Biceps brachii
- ☐ Triceps brachii
- ☐ Latissimus dorsi

Scapular Muscles

- ☐ Trapezius
- ☐ Levator scapulae
- ☐ Rhomboids

ACTIVITY 4 Range-of-Motion Tests

Instructions ➤ Ask your patient to complete active range of motion (AROM) for the movements listed. Note the available range of motion (ROM) and any discomfort.

Passive Range of Motion

After observing AROM, assess passive range of motion (PROM) for the movements listed here. Compare the results bilaterally and with the normal ROMs reported in your textbook.

	Range of Motion (Degrees)		
	Right	**Left**	**Normal**
SHOULDER			
Flexion	_____	_____	_____
Extension	_____	_____	_____
Abduction	_____	_____	_____
Adduction	_____	_____	_____
Internal rotation	_____	_____	_____
External rotation	_____	_____	_____

End-feels

PROM should include an assessment of end-feels. Provide a force at the end of the PROM and note the sensation. Record the physiological end-feel for the movement indicated, and note whether a pathological end-feel is present.

	Physiological End-feel	Pathological End-feel (If Present)
Flexion		
Extension		
Abduction		
Adduction		
Internal rotation		
External rotation		

Resisted Range of Motion

Complete resisted range of motion (RROM) for the movements listed here. Position your patient as indicated, and stabilize the joint to prevent unwanted movement. Resistive movements should include concentric, eccentric, and isometric muscle actions. Identify prime movers as you complete the assessment.

Shoulder Range of Motion and Position	Movements (Concentric, Eccentric, and Isometric)	Prime Movers
Flexion—short sitting		
Extension—lying prone		
Abduction—short sitting		
Adduction—short sitting		
Internal rotation—lying prone with 90 degrees shoulder abduction and 90 degrees elbow flexion		
External rotation—lying prone with 90 degrees shoulder abduction and 90 degrees elbow flexion		

ACTIVITY 5   Joint Stability Tests

Introduction

Injury to ligaments supporting a joint can be identified through stability tests. During these stability tests, *laxity,* or the amount of movement allowed by a joint's capsule and/or ligaments, is compared bilaterally. In addition, the *end-feel,* or sensation felt by the examiner at the limit of the stability test, is noted. Generally speaking, the end-feel during a stability test of a healthy joint is firm and definite, whereas the end-feel of an injured joint is soft and indefinite.

Instructions ➤ Provide the name for the stability test designed to test the given ligament, and then perform each test using classmates as patients. If more than one blank is included, provide alternative tests. Inherent variability of laxity exists among the healthy population. Complete the stability tests on several subjects until you have identified classmates with different grades of laxity. When two classmates with differences in laxity have been identified, you can perform the stability tests to get a better feel for a positive sign of laxity. In an actual injury assessment, this comparison would be made bilaterally.

Joint	Stability Tests
Acromioclavicular joint	
Sternoclavicular joint	
Glenohumeral joint	

Instructions ➤ Define the following grades of laxity when assessing glenohumeral glide. Perform the load-and-shift technique on several classmates, and note the grade.

Trace (0) _____

Grade I _____

Grade II _____

Grade III _____

ACTIVITY 6   Special Tests

Introduction

Certain specific injuries and conditions, such as biceps tendon pathology and impingement syndrome, require special tests that do not fit into the other assessment categories. These tests are often designed to stress a specific structure through scripted movements.

Instructions ➤ Provide the name for or describe (if there is no specific name) the special test or tests that may be used to identify the injuries and conditions listed here. Complete the special tests using your partner as the injured athlete. Describe a positive sign, and record this information in the space provided. If more than one blank is included, provide alternative tests. If there are multiple tests for the same condition, note any specific purpose for each test in the margins of the page.

Injury/Condition	Special Test	Positive Sign
Biceps tendon pathology		
Thoracic outlet syndrome		

Injury/Condition	Special Test	Positive Sign
Winging scapula	_____	_____
Impingement syndrome	_____	_____
	_____	_____
Supraspinatus pathology	_____	_____
	_____	_____
SLAP lesion	_____	_____

ACTIVITY 7   Neurologic Tests

Instructions ➤ Complete a thorough neurologic assessment for the shoulder by completing the tests outlined in the following chart. Include dermatome, myotome, and reflex testing.

Nerve Root	Dermatome	Sensory Nerve	Myotome	Motor Nerve	Reflex
C5	Lateral arm	Axillary	Shoulder abduction	Axillary	Biceps
C6	Lateral forearm/ fingers 1 and 2	Musculocu- taneous	Elbow flexion	Musculocu- taneous	Brachioradialis
C7	Third finger	Radial	Elbow extension	Radial	Triceps
C8	Medial forearm/ fingers 4 and 5	Ulnar	Finger flexion	Median/palmar interosseous	None
T1	Medial elbow	Medial brachial cutaneous	None	None	None

ACTIVITY 8   Skill Integration: Shoulder

Scenario A female javelin thrower comes to you complaining of left shoulder pain that is getting increasingly worse. She reports no distal neurologic symptoms. (You do not need to include a neurologic screen.) Demonstrate and explain your assessment of this injury. The model will not respond to your questions but will perform any actions that you request.

Optional: You have _____ minutes to complete your evaluation.

Evaluation

Name:_____   Date: _____

History				
Establishes mechanism of injury	YES	☐	NO	☐
Establishes prior history (to either shoulder)	YES	☐	NO	☐
Establishes duration of pain	YES	☐	NO	☐
Establishes location of pain	YES	☐	NO	☐
Establishes type of pain	YES	☐	NO	☐
Establishes type of symptoms (e.g., "going out")	YES	☐	NO	☐
Establishes pain/symptom pattern (e.g., night pain, after exercise)	YES	☐	NO	☐
Establishes workout pattern (e.g., significant increase in throwing)	YES	☐	NO	☐
Establishes presence/absence of other condition (e.g., spleen injury)	YES	☐	NO	☐

Inspection				
Inspects for the following:				
Swelling	YES	☐	NO	☐
Scars	YES	☐	NO	☐
Discoloration	YES	☐	NO	☐
Anterior asymmetry (e.g., atrophy, acromioclavicular [AC] joint height)	YES	☐	NO	☐
Posterior asymmetry (e.g., position of scapula, atrophy)	YES	☐	NO	☐
General posture/position of head	YES	☐	NO	☐
Compensatory movements	YES	☐	NO	☐
Performs inspection bilaterally (or states would do so)	YES	☐	NO	☐

Palpation				
Palpates for presence of the following:				
Point tenderness	YES	☐	NO	☐
Swelling	YES	☐	NO	☐
Deformity	YES	☐	NO	☐
Performs all palpation bilaterally (or states would do so)	YES	☐	NO	☐
Palpates bony and ligamentous structures:				
Sternoclavicular (SC) joint	YES	☐	NO	☐
Clavicle	YES	☐	NO	☐
AC joint	YES	☐	NO	☐
Coracoid process	YES	☐	NO	☐
Humeral head/shaft	YES	☐	NO	☐
Greater tuberosity	YES	☐	NO	☐
Bicipital groove	YES	☐	NO	☐
Spine of scapula	YES	☐	NO	☐
Scapular borders	YES	☐	NO	☐

(Continued)

Palpates soft tissue structures:

Deltoid	YES	☐	NO	☐
Pectoralis major	YES	☐	NO	☐
Supraspinatus muscle	YES	☐	NO	☐
Rotator cuff tendons/subacromial bursa (extend shoulder passively)	YES	☐	NO	☐
Infraspinatus/teres minor muscles	YES	☐	NO	☐
Biceps/biceps tendon	YES	☐	NO	☐
Triceps	YES	☐	NO	☐
Axilla	YES	☐	NO	☐
Trapezius	YES	☐	NO	☐

Range-of-Motion Testing

Response is incorrect if actions not performed correctly (i.e., proper hand placement, adequate resistance, elimination of substituting movements). GH movements: flexion/extension, abduction/adduction, internal/external rotation, horizontal flexion/extension. Scapular movements: protraction/retraction and elevation.

AROM

GH movements	YES	☐	NO	☐
Scapular movements	YES	☐	NO	☐
Cervical AROM	YES	☐	NO	☐

PROM

GH movements	YES	☐	NO	☐

RROM

GH movements	YES	☐	NO	☐
Scapular movements	YES	☐	NO	☐
Performs all tests bilaterally (or states would do so)	YES	☐	NO	☐

Ligamentous and Capsular Testing

Response is incorrect if test is performed incorrectly (i.e., proper hand position, appropriate direction and amount of stress).

Assess for sternoclavicular laxity	YES	☐	NO	☐
Assess for acromioclavicular laxity	YES	☐	NO	☐
Assess for glenohumeral laxity (posterior/inferior/anterior) (may include sulcus sign)	YES	☐	NO	☐

Special Tests

Response is incorrect if test is performed incorrectly (i.e., proper hand placement, appropriate direction and amount of stress).

Traction test	YES	☐	NO	☐
AC compression test	YES	☐	NO	☐
Empty can test (supraspinatus resistance)	YES	☐	NO	☐
Yergason test/Speed's test	YES	☐	NO	☐
Anterior apprehension test	YES	☐	NO	☐
Relocation test for anterior instability	YES	☐	NO	☐

Posterior apprehension test (may include testing in the scapular plane) ....YES ☐   NO ☐

Shoulder impingement test (with any modification) ....YES ☐   NO ☐

Drop arm test ....YES ☐   NO ☐

Yergason test ....YES ☐   NO ☐

Speed's test ....YES ☐   NO ☐

Performs all tests bilaterally (or states would do so) ....YES ☐   NO ☐

Presentation

Performs evaluation in a confident, professional manner ....YES ☐   NO ☐

Performs evaluation in a logical order ....YES ☐   NO ☐

Performs evaluation within allotted time ....YES ☐   NO ☐

TOTAL: _____ / _____

Evaluator: _____

Comments: _____

_____

ACTIVITY 9   Practical Questions

Instructions ➤   After reading the chapters in your textbook dealing with the shoulder and completing the corresponding activities, complete the following questions using your lab partner as the patient. The performance evaluation sheets that follow can be used by your instructor to grade the quality of your response to each question.

1. Name and palpate the bones and significant bony landmarks that make up the shoulder complex.

2. Perform a thorough assessment of the stability of the shoulder complex. For each test, include the name, description, and positive sign.

3 Assess AROM at the shoulder. Include normal values, and identify how you can tell if ROM is abnormal. After completing the active movements, assess PROM and identify the physiological end-feel for each anatomical movement.

4. Complete a thorough assessment of muscle function at the shoulder joint. Include a prime mover for each anatomical movement.

5. You suspect that your patient has a rotator cuff impingement involving the supraspinatus. Conduct special tests for supraspinatus function and those that would confirm an impingement syndrome. For each test, include the name, description, and positive sign.

6. Your patient complains of chronic shoulder pain and experiences pain on resisted shoulder flexion. What injury would you suspect? Conduct special tests that could be used to confirm your suspicions. For each test, include the name, description, and positive sign.

7. Complete all special tests used to identify thoracic outlet syndrome. For each test, include the name, description, and positive sign.

PERFORMANCE EVALUATION SHEETS

1. *Name and palpate the bones and significant bony landmarks that make up the shoulder complex.*

   Performance evaluation

	Name	Palpation
Sternum		
Clavicle		
Acromioclavicular (AC) joint		
Sternoclavicular (SC) joint		
Acromion process		
Coracoid process		
Scapular spine		
Superior angle		
Inferior angle		
Medial border		
Head of the humerus		
Bicipital groove		
Greater tuberosity		
Lesser tuberosity		

2. *Perform a thorough assessment of the stability of the shoulder complex. For each test, include the name, description, and positive sign.*

   Performance evaluation

	Test	Description	Positive Sign
GLENOHUMERAL JOINT			
_____ Apprehension test			
AC JOINT			
_____ Palpation			
_____ Spring test			
_____ Distraction			
SC JOINT			
_____ Palpation			
_____ Spring test			
SCAPULOTHORACIC JOINT			
_____ Wall push-up			
Bilateral comparison _____			

3. *Assess AROM at the shoulder. Include normal values, and identify how you can tell if ROM is abnormal. After completing the active movements, assess PROM and identify the physiological end-feel for each anatomical movement.*

Performance evaluation

	Normal Values	Fulcrum	Arms
Flexion	(180)		
Extension	(60)		
Internal rotation	(90)		
External rotation	(90)		
Abduction	(180)		
Adduction	(45)		

	Physiological End-feel
Flexion	
Extension	
Internal rotation	
External rotation	
Abduction	
Adduction	
Bilateral comparison	

4. *Complete a thorough assessment of muscle function at the shoulder joint. Include a prime mover for each anatomical movement.*

Performance evaluation

	Test	Prime Mover
Flexion		
Extension		
Internal rotation		
External rotation		
Abduction		
Adduction		

Active _____ Resistive _____

Isometric/breaking
point test _____ Concentric _____ Eccentric _____

Bilateral comparison _____

5. *You suspect that your patient has a rotator cuff impingement involving the supraspinatus. Conduct special tests for supraspinatus function and those that would confirm an impingement syndrome. For each test, include the name, description, and positive sign.*

Performance evaluation

	Test	Description	Positive Sign
_____ Drop arm test			
_____ Empty can test			

(Continued)

	Test	Description	Positive Sign
_____ Neer impingement test	_____	_____	_____
_____ Hawkins impingement test	_____	_____	_____
Bilateral comparison _____			

6. *Your patient complains of chronic shoulder pain and experiences pain on resisted shoulder flexion. What injury would you suspect? Conduct special tests that could be used to confirm your suspicions. For each test, include the name, description, and positive sign.*

Performance evaluation

Biceps tendinitis or tenosynovitis _____

	Test	Description	Positive Sign
_____ Speed's test	_____	_____	_____
_____ Yergason test	_____	_____	_____
Bilateral comparison _____			

7. *Complete all special tests used to identify thoracic outlet syndrome. For each test, include the name, description, and positive sign.*

Performance evaluation

	Test	Description	Positive Sign
_____ Adson's test	_____	_____	_____
_____ Allen test	_____	_____	_____
_____ Military brace position	_____	_____	_____
Bilateral comparison _____			

ANSWER KEY

Activity 4

End-feels

Flexion	Firm
Extension	Firm
Abduction	Firm
Adduction	Firm
Internal rotation	Firm
External rotation	Firm

Activity 5

Stability Tests

Acromioclavicular joint	AC compression test (spring test)
	AC traction test

Sternoclavicular joint	SC compression test (spring test)
Glenohumeral joint	Apprehension test (crank test)
	Relocation test

Activity 5   *Grades of Laxity*

Trace (0)	No translation of the humeral head
Grade I	Translation of the humeral head to the glenoid rim, but not over it
Grade II	Translation of the humeral head over the glenoid rim, but the head reduces
Grade III	The humeral head dislocates

Activity 6

Biceps tendon pathology	Yergason test	Pain and/or snapping in bicipital groove
	Speed's test	Pain in bicipital groove
Thoracic outlet syndrome	Adson's test	Radial pulse disappears
	Allen test	Radial pulse disappears
	Military brace position	Radial pulse disappears
Winging scapula	Wall push-up	Vertebral border of scapula protrudes posteriorly
Impingement syndrome	Neer impingement test	Pain near end of ROM
	Hawkins impingement test	Reproduction of impingement pain
Supraspinatus pathology	Drop arm test	Arm falls to side
	Empty can test	Weakness or pain
SLAP lesion	O'Brien test	Pain on top of shoulder or clunk

Chapter 8

Assessing the Elbow and Forearm

CHAPTER OUTLINE

Activity 6 ➤   SPECIAL TESTS

Introduction
Instructions

Activity 7 ➤   NEUROLOGIC TESTS

Instructions

Activity 8 ➤   SKILL INTEGRATION: ELBOW

Scenario
Evaluation

Activity 9 ➤   PRACTICAL QUESTIONS

Instructions

PERFORMANCE EVALUATION SHEETS
ANSWER KEY

Activity 4: End-feels
Activity 5
Activity 6

ACTIVITY 1   History

Instructions ➤   Have your partner select a common acute injury from the body part that you are studying. Ask a series of questions in an attempt to narrow the injury possibilities and guide the assessment. Your partner should provide the answers that would be likely from an athlete who sustained this injury. Record all questions and responses, and discuss your conclusions with your partner and your instructor. Repeat the process using a chronic injury.

Acute Injury

Question: _____

Response: _____

Question: _____

Response: _____

Question: _____

Response: _____

Question: _____

Response: _____

Question: _____

Response: _____

Question: _____

Response: _____

Question: _____

Response: _____

Question: _____

Response: _____

Question: _____

Response: _____

Question: _____

Response: _____

Chronic Injury

Question: _____

Response: _____

Question: _____

Response: _____

Question: _____

Response: _____

Question: _____

Response: _____

Question: _____

Response: _____

Question: _____

Response: _____

Question: _____

Response: _____

Question: _____

Response: _____

Question: _____

Response: _____

ACTIVITY 2   Inspection

Instructions ➤ Obtaining quantitative measurements often may be necessary to directly identify conditions or to identify predisposing factors that are important in the overall assessment. Complete the following measurements on your partner, and compare these measurements bilaterally, when appropriate. Also compare these measurements with other classmates and with normal values. If pathological values are found, discuss the implications for orthopedic injury and possible methods of intervention.

Carrying Angle

The *carrying angle* refers to the normal angle at the elbow when the elbow is fully extended in the anatomical position and is as follows:

- Men—10 degrees valgus
- Women—10 to 15 degrees valgus

If the carrying angle is greater than normal, *cubitus valgus* is present. If the carrying angle is less than normal, *cubitus varus* is present. An abnormal angle caused by the malunion of a humerus fracture is termed a *gunstock deformity.*

Cubital Recurvatum

The normal value for elbow extension is 0 degrees. When elbow extension is greater than 0 degrees, a deformity termed *cubital recurvatum* is present. Measure other students' elbow extension, and note extension beyond 0 degrees.

ACTIVITY 3   Palpation

Bony Palpation

Instructions ➤ Review the sections on bony anatomy in your textbook before completing this exercise. Begin by labeling the bony landmarks directly on Fig. 8–1, using the help of your textbook when needed. Develop a systematic approach so that no important structures are missed. Complete the remainder of the assignment after taking a break.

Without the aid of your textbook or skeleton, locate each bony landmark on your partner. When you have found the landmark, mark its location with a small sticker and place a check next to the landmark listed here. Use available resources (e.g., textbook, skeleton, instructor) to check the accuracy of your palpation.

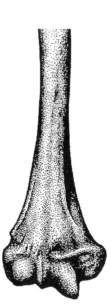

Figure 8–1   The distal humerus. (From Starkey, C, and Ryan, J: Evaluation of Orthopedic and Athletic Injuries, ed 2. FA Davis, Philadelphia, 2002, with permission.)

Lateral Aspect

☐ Lateral humeral epicondyle
☐ Radial head
☐ Capitulum

Medial Aspect

☐ Medial humeral epicondyle

Posterior Aspect

☐ Olecranon process

Soft Tissue Palpation

Instructions ➤ Review the sections on soft tissue anatomy of the elbow and forearm in your textbook before completing this exercise. Begin by locating each structure in a figure in your textbook. Develop a systematic approach so that no important structures are missed. Complete the remainder of the assignment after taking a break.

Without the aid of your textbook or skeleton, locate each structure on your partner. When you have found the landmark, mark its location with a small sticker and place a check next to the landmark listed here. For lengthy or large structures, mark a prominent portion. Use available resources (e.g., textbook, skeleton, instructor) to check the accuracy of your palpation markers.

Anterior Aspect

☐ Biceps brachii

Medial Aspect

☐ Ulnar collateral ligament
☐ Wrist flexor group

Lateral Aspect

☐ Radial collateral ligament
☐ Brachioradialis
☐ Wrist extensor group

Posterior Aspect

☐ Triceps brachii

ACTIVITY 4   Range-of-Motion Tests

Instructions ➤ Ask your patient to complete active range of motion (AROM) for the movements listed on page 117. Note the available range of motion (ROM) and any discomfort.

Passive Range of Motion

After observing AROM, assess passive range of motion (PROM) for the following movements. Compare the results bilaterally and with the normal ROMs reported in your textbook.

	Range of Motion (Degrees)		
	Right	**Left**	**Normal**
ELBOW			
Flexion	_____	_____	_____
Extension	_____	_____	_____
FOREARM			
Pronation	_____	_____	_____
Supination	_____	_____	_____

End-feels

PROM should include an assessment of end-feels. Provide a force at the end of the PROM and note the sensation. Record the physiological end-feel for the movement indicated, and note whether a pathological end-feel is present.

	Physiological End-feel	**Pathological End-feel (If Present)**
ELBOW		
Flexion	_____	_____
Extension	_____	_____
FOREARM		
Pronation	_____	_____
Supination	_____	_____

Resisted Range of Motion

Complete resisted range of motion (RROM) for the movements listed here. Position your patient as indicated, and stabilize the joint to prevent unwanted movement. Resistive movements should include concentric, eccentric, and isometric muscle actions. Identify prime movers as you complete the assessment.

Range of Motion and Position	Movements (Concentric, Eccentric, and Isometric)	Prime Movers
ELBOW		
Flexion—short sitting	_____	_____
Extension—lying prone with 90 degrees of shoulder abduction and 90 degrees of elbow flexion	_____	_____

(Continued)

Range of Motion and Position	Movements (Concentric, Eccentric, and Isometric)	Prime Movers
FOREARM		
Pronation—short sitting with 90 degrees of elbow flexion	_____	_____
Supination—short sitting with 90 degrees of elbow flexion	_____	_____

ACTIVITY 5   Joint Stability

Introduction

Injury to ligaments supporting a joint can be identified through stability tests. During these stability tests, *laxity,* or the amount of movement allowed by a joint's capsule and ligaments, is compared bilaterally. In addition, the *end-feel,* or sensation felt by the examiner at the limit of the stability test, is noted. Generally speaking, the end-feel during a stability test of a healthy joint is firm and definite, whereas the end-feel of an injured joint is soft and indefinite.

Instructions ➤ Provide the name for the stability test designed to test the given ligament, and then perform each test using classmates as patients. If more than one blank is included, provide alternative tests. Inherent variability of laxity exists among the healthy population. Complete the stability tests on several subjects until you have identified classmates with different grades of laxity. When two classmates with differences in laxity have been identified, you can perform the stability tests to get a better feel for a positive sign of laxity. In an actual injury assessment, this comparison would be made bilaterally.

Ligament	Stability Test
Ulnar collateral ligament (UCL)	_____
Radial collateral ligament (RCL)	_____

ACTIVITY 6   Special Tests

Introduction

Certain specific injuries and conditions, such as epicondylitis, require special tests that do not fit into the other assessment categories. These tests are often designed to stress a specific structure through scripted movements.

Instructions ➤ Provide the name for or describe (if there is no specific name) the special test or tests that may be used to identify the injuries and conditions listed here. Complete the special tests using your partner as the injured athlete. Describe a positive sign, and record this information in the space provided. If more than one blank is included, provide alternative tests.

Injury/Condition	Special Test	Positive Sign
Lateral epicondylitis	_____	_____
Medial epicondylitis	_____	_____
Radial tunnel syndrome	_____	_____

ACTIVITY 7   Neurologic Tests

Instructions ➤   Complete a thorough neurologic assessment for the elbow and forearm by completing the tests outlined in the following chart. Include dermatome, myotome, and reflex testing.

Nerve Root	Dermatome	Sensory Nerve	Myotome	Motor Nerve	Reflex
C6	Lateral forearm; first and second fingers	Musculocutaneous	Elbow flexion	Musculocutaneous	Brachioradialis
C7	Third finger	Radial	Elbow extension	Radial	Triceps
C8	Medial forearm; fourth and fifth fingers	Ulnar	Finger flexion	Median/palmar interosseous	None
T1	Medial elbow	Medial brachial cutaneous	None	None	None

ACTIVITY 8   Skill Integration: Elbow

Scenario   A right-handed Little League baseball pitcher comes to an injury screening complaining of right elbow pain that is increasing as the season progresses. Demonstrate and explain your assessment of this injury. The model will not respond to your questions but will perform any actions that you request.

Optional: You have _____ minutes to complete your evaluation.

Evaluation

Name: _____   Date: _____

History

Establishes mechanism of injury	YES	☐	NO	☐
Establishes pitching history (i.e., number of pitches, frequency of throwing)	YES	☐	NO	☐
Establishes type of pain	YES	☐	NO	☐
Establishes location of pain	YES	☐	NO	☐
Establishes presence/absence of neurologic signs and symptoms	YES	☐	NO	☐
Establishes pain pattern	YES	☐	NO	☐
Establishes prior history	YES	☐	NO	☐
Establishes age of athlete	YES	☐	NO	☐

Inspection

Inspects for the following:

Swelling	YES	☐	NO	☐
Discoloration	YES	☐	NO	☐
Deformity (i.e., bursitis)	YES	☐	NO	☐
Carrying angle	YES	☐	NO	☐
Scars	YES	☐	NO	☐
States that inspection would occur bilaterally	YES	☐	NO	☐

Palpation

Palpates for the following:

Point tenderness	YES	☐	NO	☐
Deformity	YES	☐	NO	☐
Swelling	YES	☐	NO	☐
Temperature change	YES	☐	NO	☐
Performs all palpation bilaterally (or states would do so)	YES	☐	NO	☐

Palpates bony and ligamentous structures:

Humerus	YES	☐	NO	☐
Medial epicondyle	YES	☐	NO	☐
Radial collateral ligament	YES	☐	NO	☐
Radial head	YES	☐	NO	☐
Lateral epicondyle	YES	☐	NO	☐
Lateral collateral ligament	YES	☐	NO	☐
Olecranon process	YES	☐	NO	☐

Palpates other soft tissues:

Wrist flexor group	YES	☐	NO	☐
Wrist extensor group	YES	☐	NO	☐
Biceps tendon	YES	☐	NO	☐
Ulnar nerve	YES	☐	NO	☐

Triceps tendon		YES	☐	NO	☐
Olecranon bursa		YES	☐	NO	☐

Range-of-Motion Testing

Response is incorrect if all motions (elbow flexion/extension, forearm supination/pronation, and wrist flexion/extension) are not included. Action must be performed correctly (i.e., proper hand placement, adequate resistance).

Evaluates AROM		YES	☐	NO	☐
Evaluates PROM		YES	☐	NO	☐
Evaluates RROM		YES	☐	NO	☐
Performs all tests bilaterally (or states would do so)		YES	☐	NO	☐

Ligamentous and Capsular Testing

Response is incorrect if test is not performed correctly (i.e., proper hand placement, appropriate direction and amount of stress).

Valgus stress test in full extension		YES	☐	NO	☐
Valgus stress in 30 degrees of flexion		YES	☐	NO	☐
Varus stress test in full extension		YES	☐	NO	☐
Varus stress in 30 degrees of flexion		YES	☐	NO	☐
Performs all tests bilaterally (or states would do so)		YES	☐	NO	☐

Special Tests

Response is incorrect if test is not performed correctly (i.e., proper hand position, appropriate direction and amount of stress).

Tennis elbow test		YES	☐	NO	☐
Tinel's sign (ulnar nerve)		YES	☐	NO	☐

Neurologic Examination

Must bilaterally assess motor and sensory function for full credit.

Ulnar nerve		YES	☐	NO	☐
Radial nerve		YES	☐	NO	☐
Median nerve		YES	☐	NO	☐

Presentation

Performs evaluation in a confident, professional manner		YES	☐	NO	☐
Performs evaluation in a logical order		YES	☐	NO	☐
Performs evaluation within allotted time		YES	☐	NO	☐

TOTAL: _____ / _____

Evaluator: _____

Comments: _____

_____

_____

ACTIVITY 9   Practical Questions

Instructions ➤   After reading the chapters in your textbook dealing with the elbow and forearm and completing the corresponding activities, complete the following questions using your lab partner as the patient. The performance evaluation sheets that follow can be used by your instructor to grade the quality of your response to each question.

1. Name and palpate the bones and significant bony landmarks that make up the elbow, forearm, wrist, and hand.

2. Assess AROM at the elbow and forearm. Include normal values, and identify how you can tell if ROM is abnormal. After completing the active movements, assess PROM and identify the physiological end-feel for each anatomical movement.

3. Complete a thorough assessment of RROM at the elbow and forearm. Include a prime mover for each anatomical movement.

PERFORMANCE EVALUATION SHEETS

1. *Name and palpate the bones and significant bony landmarks that make up the elbow, forearm, wrist, and hand.*

Performance evaluation

	Name	Palpation
Medial humeral epicondyle		
Lateral humeral epicondyle		
Olecranon process		
Radial head		
Capitulum		
Ulnar styloid process		
Distal radial styloid process		
Scaphoid (navicular)		
Pisiform		
Trapezium		
Lunate		
Metacarpals		
Phalanges (proximal, medial, distal)		

2. *Assess AROM at the elbow and forearm. Include normal values, and identify how you can tell if ROM is abnormal. After completing the active movements, assess PROM and identify the physiological end-feel for each anatomical movement.*

Performance evaluation

	Normal Values	Goniometer	Fulcrum	Arms
ELBOW				
Flexion	_____	_____	_____	_____
Extension	_____	_____	_____	_____
FOREARM				
Pronation	_____	_____	_____	_____
Supination	_____	_____	_____	_____

Physiological End-feel	
ELBOW	
Flexion	_____
Extension	_____
FOREARM	
Flexion	_____
Extension	_____
Bilateral comparison	_____

3. *Complete a thorough assessment of RROM at the elbow and forearm. Include a prime mover for each anatomical movement.*

Performance evaluation

	Test	Prime Mover
ELBOW		
Flexion	_____	_____
Extension	_____	_____
FOREARM		
Pronation	_____	_____
Supination	_____	_____

Active _____ Resistive _____

Isometric/breaking
point test _____ Concentric _____ Eccentric _____

Bilateral comparison _____

ANSWER KEY

Activity 4

	End-feels
Flexion	Soft
Extension	Hard
Pronation	Hard or firm
Supination	Firm

Activity 5

Ulnar collateral ligament (UCL)	Valgus stress test
Radial collateral ligament (RCL)	Varus stress test

Activity 6

Lateral epicondylitis	Tennis elbow test	Lateral epicondyle pain
Medial epicondylitis	Resisted wrist flexion	Medial epicondyle pain
Radial tunnel syndrome	Resisted supination and middle finger extension	Radiating pain

Chapter 9

Assessing the Wrist and Hand

CHAPTER OUTLINE

ACTIVITY 1   History

Instructions ➤ Have your partner select a common acute injury from the body part that you are studying. Ask a series of questions in an attempt to narrow the injury possibilities and guide the assessment. Your partner should provide the answers that would be likely from an athlete who sustained this injury. Record all questions and responses, and discuss your conclusions with your partner and your instructor. Repeat the process using a chronic injury.

Acute Injury

Question: _____

Response: _____

Question: _____

Response: _____

Question: _____

Response: _____

Question: _____

Response: _____

Question: _____

Response: _____

Question: _____

Response: _____

Question: _____

Response: _____

Question: _____

Response: _____

Question: _____

Response: _____

Question: _____

Response: _____

Chronic Injury

Question: _____

Response: _____

Question: _____

Response: _____

Question: _____

Response: _____

Question: _____

Response: _____

Question: _____

Response: _____

Question: _____

Response: _____

Question: _____

Response: _____

Question: _____

Response: _____

Question: _____

Response: _____

Question: _____

Response: _____

ACTIVITY 2   Inspection

Instructions ➤ Define the deformities, abnormalities, and conditions listed here. Inspect your partner's lower extremity to identify each condition. Inspect other students until each of the conditions has been found. If a condition is not found within the class population, find a photograph of the deformity in your textbook.

Murphy's sign _____

Volkmann's ischemic contractures _____

Trigger finger _____

Boutonniere deformity _____

Mallet finger _____

Jersey finger _____

ACTIVITY 3 Palpation

Bony Palpation

Instructions ➤ Review the sections on bony anatomy in your textbook before completing this exercise. Begin by labeling the bony landmarks directly on Fig. 9–1, using the help of your textbook when needed. Develop a systematic approach so that no important structures are missed. Complete the remainder of the assignment after taking a break.

Without the aid of your textbook or skeleton, locate each bony landmark on your partner. When you have found the landmark, mark its position with a small sticker and place a check next to the landmark listed here. Use available resources (e.g., textbook, skeleton, instructor) to check the accuracy of your palpation.

- ☐ Ulnar styloid process
- ☐ Radial shaft
- ☐ Distal radial styloid process
- ☐ Carpals (proximal row)
  - ☐ Scaphoid (navicular)
  - ☐ Lunate
  - ☐ Triquetrum
  - ☐ Pisiform
- ☐ Carpal (distal row)
  - ☐ Trapezium
  - ☐ Trapezoid
  - ☐ Capitate
  - ☐ Hamate
- ☐ Metacarpals
- ☐ Proximal, middle, and distal phalanx

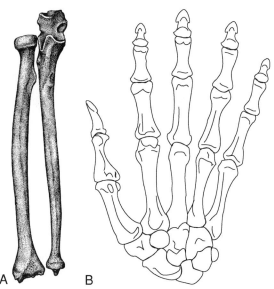

Figure 9–1 Bony anatomy of the wrist and hand. *(A)* Radius and ulna. *(B)* Wrist and hand. (From Starkey, C, and Ryan, J: Evaluation of Orthopedic and Athletic Injuries, ed 2. FA Davis, Philadelphia, 2002, with permission.)

A   B

Soft Tissue Palpation

Instructions ➤ Review the sections on soft tissue anatomy of the wrist and hand in your textbook before completing this exercise. Begin by locating each structure on a figure in your textbook. Develop a systematic approach so that no important structures are missed. Complete the remainder of the assignment after taking a break.

Without the aid of your textbook or skeleton, locate each structure on your partner. When you have found the landmark, mark its location with a small sticker and place a check next to the landmark listed here. For lengthy or large structures, mark a prominent portion. Use available resources (e.g., textbook, skeleton, instructor) to check the accuracy of your palpation markers.

Wrist: Anteromedial Aspect

☐ Ulnar collateral ligament
☐ Flexor carpi ulnaris
☐ Flexor digitorum profundus
☐ Palmaris longus
☐ Flexor carpi radialis

Wrist: Posterolateral Aspect

☐ Radial collateral ligament
☐ Extensor carpi radialis longus
☐ Extensor carpi radialis brevis
☐ Extensor digitorum
☐ Extensor carpi ulnaris
☐ Thumb extensors

Hand

☐ Collateral ligament of metacarpophalangeal (MCP) joints
☐ Collateral ligament of interphalangeal joints
☐ Thenar compartment
☐ Thenar web space
☐ Central compartment
☐ Hypothenar compartment

ACTIVITY 4   Range-of-Motion Tests

Instructions ➤ Ask your patient to complete active range of motion (AROM) for the movements listed on page 130. Note the available range of motion (ROM) and any discomfort.

Passive Range of Motion

After observing AROM, assess passive range of motion (PROM) for the following movements. Compare the results bilaterally and with the normal ROMs reported in your textbook.

	Range of Motion (Degrees)		
	Right	**Left**	**Normal**
WRIST			
Flexion	_____	_____	_____
Extension	_____	_____	_____
Radial deviation	_____	_____	_____
Ulnar deviation	_____	_____	_____
THUMB (CARPOMETACARPAL JOINT)			
Flexion	_____	_____	_____
Extension	_____	_____	_____
Abduction	_____	_____	_____
Adduction	_____	_____	_____
THUMB (INTERPHALANGEAL JOINT)			
Flexion	_____	_____	_____
Extension	_____	_____	_____
FINGER (MCP JOINT)			
Flexion	_____	_____	_____
Extension	_____	_____	_____
Abduction	_____	_____	_____
Adduction	_____	_____	_____
FINGER (PROXIMAL INTERPHALANGEAL [PIP] JOINT)			
Flexion	_____	_____	_____
Extension	_____	_____	_____
FINGER (DISTAL INTERPHALANGEAL [DIP] JOINT)			
Flexion	_____	_____	_____
Extension	_____	_____	_____

End-feels

PROM should include an assessment of end-feels. Provide a force at the end of the PROM and note the sensation. Record the physiological end-feel for the movement indicated, and note whether a pathological end-feel is present.

	Physiological End-feel	**Pathological End-feel (If Present)**
WRIST		
Flexion	_____	_____
Extension	_____	_____

	Physiological End-feel	Pathological End-feel (If Present)
Radial deviation	_____	_____
Ulnar deviation	_____	_____
THUMB (CARPOMETACARPAL JOINT)		
Flexion	_____	_____
Extension	_____	_____
Abduction	_____	_____
Adduction	_____	_____
THUMB (INTERPHALANGEAL JOINT)		
Flexion	_____	_____
Extension	_____	_____
FINGER (MCP JOINT)		
Flexion	_____	_____
Extension	_____	_____
Abduction	_____	_____
Adduction	_____	_____
FINGER (PIP JOINT)		
Flexion	_____	_____
Extension	_____	_____
FINGER (DIP JOINT)		
Flexion	_____	_____
Extension	_____	_____

Resisted Range of Motion

Complete resisted range of motion (RROM) for the movements listed here. Position your patient as indicated, and stabilize the joint to prevent unwanted movement. Resistive movements should include concentric, eccentric, and isometric muscle actions. Identify prime movers as you complete the assessment.

Range of Motion and Position	Movement (Concentric, Eccentric, and Isometric)	Prime Movers
WRIST		
Flexion	_____	_____
Extension	_____	_____
Radial deviation	_____	_____
Ulnar deviation	_____	_____

(Continued)

Range of Motion and Position	Movement (Concentric, Eccentric, and Isometric)	Prime Movers
THUMB (CARPOMETACARPAL JOINT)		
Flexion		
Extension		
Abduction		
Adduction		
THUMB (INTERPHALANGEAL JOINT)		
Flexion		
Extension		
FINGER (MCP JOINT)		
Flexion		
Extension		
Abduction		
Adduction		
FINGER (PIP JOINT)		
Flexion		
Extension		
FINGER (DIP JOINT)		
Flexion		
Extension		

ACTIVITY 5　Joint Stability Tests

Introduction

Injury to ligaments supporting a joint can be identified through stability tests. During these stability tests, *laxity*, or the amount of movement allowed by a joint's capsule and ligaments, is compared bilaterally. In addition, the *end-feel*, or sensation felt by the examiner at the limit of the stability test, is noted. Generally speaking, the end-feel during a stability test of a healthy joint is firm and definite, whereas the end-feel of an injured joint is soft and indefinite.

Instructions ➤ Provide the name for the stability test designed to test the given ligament, and then perform each test using classmates as patients. If more than one blank is included, provide alternative tests. Inherent variability of laxity exists among the healthy population. Complete the stability tests on several subjects until you have identified classmates with different grades of laxity. When two classmates with differences in laxity have been identified, you can perform the stability tests to get a better feel for a positive sign of laxity. In an actual injury assessment, this comparison would be made bilaterally.

After completing the assignment, discuss with your partner any joint position changes that should be performed before the stability test (e.g., flexion, rotation). Discuss the purpose for these changes in joint position.

Ligaments	Stability Tests
WRIST	
Volar ligaments	
Dorsal ligaments	
Ulnar collateral ligament	
Radial collateral ligament	
HAND	
Ulnar collateral ligaments (MCP, PIP, DIP joints)	
Radial collateral ligament (MCP, PIP, DIP joints)	
Volar plate (MCP, PIP, DIP joints)	

ACTIVITY 6   Special Tests

Introduction

Certain specific injuries and conditions, such as carpal tunnel syndrome, require special tests that do not fit into the other assessment categories. These tests are often designed to stress a specific structure through scripted movements.

Instructions ➤ Provide the name for or describe (if there is no specific name) the special test or tests that may be used to identify the injuries and conditions listed here. Complete the special tests using your partner as the injured athlete. Describe a positive sign, and record this information in the space provided. If more than one blank is included, provide alternative tests.

Injury/Condition	Special Test	Positive Sign
de Quervain's disease		
Carpal tunnel syndrome		

ACTIVITY 7   Neurologic Tests

Instructions ➤ Complete a thorough neurologic assessment for the wrist and hand by completing the tests outlined in the following chart. Include dermatome, myotome, and reflex testing.

Nerve Root	Dermatome	Sensory Nerve	Myotome	Motor Nerve	Reflex
C6	Lateral forearm; first and second fingers	Musculocutaneous	Elbow flexion	Musculocutaneous	Brachioradialis
C7	Third finger	Radial	Elbow extension	Radial	Triceps
C8	Medial forearm; fourth and fifth fingers	Ulnar	Finger flexion	Median/palmar interosseous	None
T1	Medial elbow	Medial brachial cutaneous	None	None	None

ACTIVITY 8   Skill Integration: Wrist and Hand

Scenario   A member of the crew (rowing) team comes to you complaining of right wrist pain that has been present for the past month. Demonstrate and explain your assessment of this injury. The model will not respond to your questions but will perform any actions that you request.

Optional: You have _____ minutes to complete your evaluation.

Evaluation

Name: _____   Date: _____

History				
Establishes any specific mechanism of injury	YES	☐	NO	☐
Establishes prior history of wrist/hand injury	YES	☐	NO	☐
Establishes prior injury	YES	☐	NO	☐
Establishes location of pain	YES	☐	NO	☐
Establishes type of pain	YES	☐	NO	☐
Establishes pain pattern	YES	☐	NO	☐
Establishes presence or absence of crepitus	YES	☐	NO	☐
Establishes progression of symptoms	YES	☐	NO	☐
Establishes presence or absence of pain elsewhere on the body	YES	☐	NO	☐
Establishes presence or absence of neurologic symptoms	YES	☐	NO	☐

Inspection				
Inspects for the following:				
Swelling	YES	☐	NO	☐
Discoloration	YES	☐	NO	☐
States that observation occurs bilaterally	YES	☐	NO	☐

Palpation				
Palpates for the presence of the following:				
Point tenderness	YES	☐	NO	☐
Swelling	YES	☐	NO	☐
Crepitus	YES	☐	NO	☐
Performs palpation bilaterally (or states would do so)	YES	☐	NO	☐
Palpates bony and ligamentous structures:				
Radial styloid process	YES	☐	NO	☐
Scaphoid	YES	☐	NO	☐
Lunate	YES	☐	NO	☐
Triquetrum	YES	☐	NO	☐
Pisiform	YES	☐	NO	☐
Trapezium	YES	☐	NO	☐
Trapezoid	YES	☐	NO	☐
Hamate	YES	☐	NO	☐
Ulnar styloid process	YES	☐	NO	☐
Phalanges	YES	☐	NO	☐
Metacarpal bones	YES	☐	NO	☐
Palpates other soft tissues:				
Thenar eminence	YES	☐	NO	☐
Hypothenar eminence	YES	☐	NO	☐

(Continued)

Extensor pollicis longus	YES ☐	NO ☐
Abductor pollicis longus	YES ☐	NO ☐
Extensor pollicis longus	YES ☐	NO ☐
First metacarpophalangeal (MCP) joint	YES ☐	NO ☐
Carpal tunnel	YES ☐	NO ☐

Range-of-Motion Testing

Response is incorrect if all actions (wrist flexion/extension, thumb abduction/adduction, thumb flexion/extension, opposition, ulnar and radial deviation, pronation, supination) are not included. Action must be performed correctly (i.e., proper hand placement, adequate resistance, elimination of substituting movements).

Evaluates wrist, hand, and forearm AROM	YES ☐	NO ☐
Evaluates wrist, hand, and forearm PROM	YES ☐	NO ☐
Evaluates wrist, hand, and forearm RROM	YES ☐	NO ☐
Performs ROM bilaterally (or states would do so)	YES ☐	NO ☐

Ligamentous and Capsular Testing

Response is incorrect if test is not performed correctly (i.e., proper hand placement, appropriate direction and amount of stress).

Stress ulnar collateral ligament (UCL)–first MCP	YES ☐	NO ☐
Valgus stress test–radiocarpal joint	YES ☐	NO ☐
Varus stress test–radiocarpal joint	YES ☐	NO ☐
Glide testing of wrist	YES ☐	NO ☐

Special Tests

Response is incorrect if test is not performed correctly (i.e., proper hand position, appropriate direction and amount of stress).

Tinel's sign (median nerve)	YES ☐	NO ☐
Phalen's test	YES ☐	NO ☐
Finkelstein's test	YES ☐	NO ☐

Neurologic Tests

Must assess motor and sensory function for full credit.

Radial nerve	YES ☐	NO ☐
Median nerve	YES ☐	NO ☐
Ulnar nerve	YES ☐	NO ☐

Presentation

Performs evaluation in a confident, professional manner	YES ☐	NO ☐
Performs evaluation in a logical sequence	YES ☐	NO ☐
Performs evaluation within allotted time	YES ☐	NO ☐

TOTAL: _____ / _____

Evaluator: _____

Comments: _____

_____

_____

ACTIVITY 9   Practical Questions

Instructions ➤   After reading the chapters in your textbook dealing with the wrist and hand, and completing the corresponding activities, complete the following questions using your lab partner as the patient. The performance evaluation sheets that follow can be used by your instructor to grade the quality of your response to each question.

1. Assess AROM at the wrist and hand. Include normal values, and identify how you can tell if ROM is abnormal. After completing the active movements, assess PROM and identify the physiological end-feel for each anatomical movement.

2. Complete a thorough assessment of RROM at the wrist and hand. Include a prime mover for each anatomical movement.

PERFORMANCE EVALUATION SHEETS

1. *Assess AROM at the wrist and hand. Include normal values, and identify how you can tell if ROM is abnormal. After completing the active movements, assess PROM and identify the physiological end-feel for each anatomical movement.*

Performance evaluation

	Normal Values	Goniometer	Fulcrum	Arms
WRIST				
Flexion	_____	_____	_____	_____
Extension	_____	_____	_____	_____
Radial deviation	_____	_____	_____	_____
Ulnar deviation	_____	_____	_____	_____
THUMB (CARPOMETACARPAL JOINT)				
Flexion	_____	_____	_____	_____
Extension	_____	_____	_____	_____
Abduction	_____	_____	_____	_____
Adduction	_____	_____	_____	_____
THUMB (INTERPHALANGEAL JOINT)				
Flexion	_____	_____	_____	_____
Extension	_____	_____	_____	_____
FINGER (METACARPOPHALANGEAL JOINT)				
Flexion	_____	_____	_____	_____
Extension	_____	_____	_____	_____
Abduction	_____	_____	_____	_____
Adduction	_____	_____	_____	_____

(Continued)

	Normal Values	Goniometer	Fulcrum	Arms

FINGER (PROXIMAL INTERPHALANGEAL JOINT)

Flexion	_____	_____	_____	_____
Extension	_____	_____	_____	_____

FINGER (DISTAL INTERPHALANGEAL JOINT)

Flexion	_____	_____	_____	_____
Extension	_____	_____	_____	_____

Physiological End-feel

WRIST

Flexion	_____
Extension	_____
Radial deviation	_____
Ulnar deviation	_____

THUMB (CARPOMETACARPAL JOINT)

Flexion	_____
Extension	_____
Abduction	_____
Adduction	_____

THUMB (INTERPHALANGEAL JOINT)

Flexion	_____
Extension	_____

FINGER (METACARPOPHALANGEAL JOINT)

Flexion	_____
Extension	_____
Abduction	_____
Adduction	_____

FINGER (PROXIMAL INTERPHALANGEAL JOINT)

Flexion	_____
Extension	_____

FINGER (DISTAL INTERPHALANGEAL JOINT)

Flexion	_____
Extension	_____
Bilateral comparison	_____

2. *Complete a thorough assessment of RROM at the wrist and hand. Include a prime mover for each anatomical movement.*

Performance evaluation

	Test	Prime Mover

WRIST

	Test	Prime Mover
Flexion	_____	_____
Extension	_____	_____
Radial deviation	_____	_____
Ulnar deviation	_____	_____

THUMB (CARPOMETACARPAL JOINT)

	Test	Prime Mover
Flexion	_____	_____
Extension	_____	_____
Abduction	_____	_____
Adduction	_____	_____

THUMB (INTERPHALANGEAL JOINT)

	Test	Prime Mover
Flexion	_____	_____
Extension	_____	_____

FINGER (METACARPOPHALANGEAL JOINT)

	Test	Prime Mover
Flexion	_____	_____
Extension	_____	_____
Abduction	_____	_____
Adduction	_____	_____

FINGER (PROXIMAL INTERPHALANGEAL JOINT)

	Test	Prime Mover
Flexion	_____	_____
Extension	_____	_____

FINGER (DISTAL INTERPHALANGEAL JOINT)

	Test	Prime Mover
Flexion	_____	_____
Extension	_____	_____

Active _____   Resistive _____

Isometric/breaking
point test _____   Concentric _____   Eccentric _____

Bilateral comparison _____

ANSWER KEY

Activity 4   *End-feels*

WRIST

Flexion	Firm
Extension	Usually soft, sometimes hard
Radial deviation	Usually soft, sometimes hard
Ulnar deviation	Firm

THUMB (CARPOMETACARPAL JOINT)

Flexion	Soft or firm
Extension	Firm
Abduction	Firm
Adduction	Soft

THUMB (INTERPHALANGEAL JOINT)

Flexion	Usually firm, sometimes hard
Extension	Firm

FINGER (MCP JOINT)

Flexion	Hard or firm
Extension	Firm
Abduction	Firm
Adduction	Firm

FINGER (PIP JOINT)

Flexion	Usually hard, sometimes soft or firm
Extension	Firm

FINGER (DIP JOINT)

Flexion	Firm
Extension	Firm

Activity 5

WRIST

Volar ligaments	Passive wrist extension
Dorsal ligaments	Passive wrist flexion
Ulnar collateral ligament	Valgus stress test
Radial collateral ligament	Varus stress test

HAND

Ulnar collateral ligaments (MCP, PIP, DIP joints)	Valgus stress test	
Radial collateral ligament (MCP, PIP, DIP joints)	Varus stress test	
Volar plate (MCP, PIP, DIP joints)	Passive extension	

Activity 6

de Quervain's disease	Finkelstein's test	Increased pain with thumb extension
Carpal tunnel syndrome	Phalen's test	Paresthesia in distribution of median nerve
	Tinel's test	Paresthesia in distribution of median nerve

Chapter 10

Assessing the Head

ACTIVITY 1   History

Instructions ➤   Have your partner select a common acute injury from the body part that you are studying. Ask a series of questions in an attempt to narrow the injury possibilities and guide the assessment. Your partner should provide the answers that would be likely from an athlete who sustained this injury. Record all questions and responses, and discuss your conclusions with your partner and your instructor. Be sure to include questions that will identify the presence of either retrograde or anterograde amnesia.

Acute Injury

Question: _____

Response: _____

Question: _____

Response: _____

Question: _____

Response: _____

Question: _____

Response: _____

Question: _____

Response: _____

Question: _____

Response: _____

Question: _____

Response: _____

Question: _____

Response: _____

Question: _____

Response: _____

Question: _____

Response: _____

ACTIVITY 2   Inspection

Instructions ➤   Inspection of the head primarily involves a close look at the bony structures, as well as the eyes, ears, and nose. Complete the following inspection, using your partner as a model, and place a mark next to the area as the inspection is completed. Describe any positive signs of injury, including any specific areas addressed here.

☐ Inspect the skull.
   ☐ Describe Battle's sign.
      ☐ What is the implication?

☐ Inspect the face.
   ☐ Describe "raccoon eyes."
      ☐ What is the implication?

☐ Inspect the nose and ears for deformity or bleeding.
   ☐ If fluid is leaking from the nose or ear, describe the test that can be used to determine whether the fluid contains cerebrospinal fluid.

☐ Inspect the eyes.
   ☐ Note any nystagmus (involuntary cyclical movement).
      ☐ What is the implication?
   ☐ Observe pupil size (equal or unequal).
      ☐ What is the implication if unequal?

ACTIVITY 3   Neurologic Tests

Instructions ➤   Identify the name and the major functions of each of the cranial nerves. Complete a thorough neurologic assessment of each cranial nerve, supplying the test used to assess the function in the blank provided.

Number	Name	Function(s)	Test
I	_____	_____	_____
II	_____	_____	_____
III	_____	_____	_____
IV	_____	_____	_____
V	_____	_____	_____
VI	_____	_____	_____
VII	_____	_____	_____
VIII	_____	_____	_____
IX	_____	_____	_____
X	_____	_____	_____
XI	_____	_____	_____
XII	_____	_____	_____

ACTIVITY 4   Practical Questions

Instructions ➤   After reading the chapters in your textbook dealing with the head and completing the corresponding activities, complete the following question using your lab partner as the patient. The performance evaluation sheets that follow can be used by your instructor to grade the quality of your response to the question.

1. Your patient has sustained a significant head injury, and you suspect possible damage to the cranial nerves. Name the cranial nerves in numerical order, and perform a single test to assess the function of each nerve.

PERFORMANCE EVALUATION SHEETS

1. *Your patient has sustained a significant head injury, and you suspect possible damage to the cranial nerves. Name the cranial nerves in numerical order, and perform a single test to assess the function of each nerve.*

Performance evaluation

_____ Olfactory	Smell _____	Identify odor _____
_____ Optic	Visual acuity _____	Number of fingers _____
	Visual field _____	Peripheral vision _____
_____ Oculomotor	Pupillary react _____	Penlight _____

_____ Trochlear	Upward eye movement _____	Follow finger _____
_____ Trigeminal	Facial sensations _____	Touch face _____
	Motor _____	Resist closing mouth _____
_____ Abducens	Lateral eye movement _____	Follow finger _____
_____ Facial	Facial expression _____	Smile _____
	Taste _____	Identify tastes _____
_____ Vestibulocochlear	Hearing _____	Identify sounds _____
	Equilibrium _____	Romberg's _____
_____ Glossopharyngeal	Swallowing _____	Swallow _____
	Taste _____	Identify tastes _____
_____ Vagus	Gag reflex _____	Gag reflex _____
_____ Accessory	Neck strength _____	Resist shoulder shrug or turn head _____
_____ Hypoglossal	Tongue movement _____	Resist tongue movement _____

ANSWER KEY

Activity 3

I Olfactory	Smell	Identify odor
II Optic	Visual acuity	Identify number of fingers
	Visual field	Check peripheral vision
III Oculomotor	Pupillary react	Shine penlight
IV Trochlear	Upward eye movement	Follow finger
V Trigeminal	Facial sensations	Touch face
	Motor function	Resist closing mouth
VI Abducens	Lateral eye movement	Follow finger
VII Facial	Facial expression	Smile
	Taste	Identify tastes
VIII Vestibulocochlear	Hearing	Identify sounds
	Equilibrium	Check Romberg's
IX Glossopharyngeal	Swallowing	Swallow
	Taste	Identify tastes
X Vagus	Gag reflex	Elicit gag reflex
XI Accessory	Neck strength	Resist shoulder shrug
XII Hypoglossal	Tongue movement	Resist tongue movement

Chapter 11

Assessing Nonorthopedic Conditions

Activity 8 ➤   FACE AND RELATED STRUCTURES: HISTORY

Instructions
    Acute injury
    Chronic injury

Activity 9 ➤   FACE AND RELATED STRUCTURES: INSPECTION

Instructions
    Ear
    Nose
    Face and jaw
Instructions
Instructions
    Ear
    Nose

Activity 10 ➤   FACE AND RELATED STRUCTURES: PALPATION

Instructions

Activity 11 ➤   FACE AND RELATED STRUCTURES: SPECIAL TESTS

Introduction
Instructions

Activity 12 ➤   ENVIRONMENTAL CONDITIONS: HISTORY

Instructions

Activity 13 ➤   ENVIRONMENTAL CONDITIONS: INSPECTION AND PALPATION

Instructions

Activity 14 ➤   ENVIRONMENTAL CONDITIONS: SLING PSYCHROMETER

Instructions

Activity 15 ➤   CARDIOPULMONARY CONDITIONS: HISTORY

Instructions

Activity 16 ➤   CARDIOPULMONARY CONDITIONS: INSPECTION AND PALPATION

Instructions
    Unconscious athlete
    Conscious athlete

Activity 17 ➤   SKILL INTEGRATION: CARDIOPULMONARY CONDITION

Scenario
Evaluation

Activity 18 ➤   PRACTICAL QUESTIONS

Instructions

PERFORMANCE EVALUATION SHEETS

ANSWER KEY

Activity 2: Abdomen
Activity 3
Activity 11
Activity 13

ACTIVITY 1   Thorax and Abdomen: History

Instructions ➤ Have your partner select a medical condition or injury of the thorax that was discussed in your textbook. Ask a series of questions in an attempt to narrow the condition or injury possibilities and guide the assessment. Your partner should provide the answers that would be likely from an athlete who sustained this condition or injury. Record all questions and responses, and discuss your conclusions with your partner and instructor. Repeat this process using a medical condition or injury for the abdomen.

Thorax

Question: _____
Response: _____

Question: _____
Response: _____

Question: _____
Response: _____

Question: _____
Response: _____

Question: _____
Response: _____

Question: _____
Response: _____

Question: _____
Response: _____

Question: _____
Response: _____

Question: _____
Response: _____

Question: _____
Response: _____

Question: _____
Response: _____

Abdomen

Question: _____
Response: _____

Question: _____

Response: _____

Question: _____

Response: _____

Question: _____

Response: _____

Question: _____

Response: _____

Question: _____

Response: _____

Question: _____

Response: _____

Question: _____

Response: _____

Question: _____

Response: _____

Question: _____

Response: _____

ACTIVITY 2   Thorax and Abdomen: Palpation, Auscultation, and Percussion

Instructions ➤   This exercise is designed to improve your palpation, auscultation, and percussion skills. Complete the following using your partner as a model, placing a check next to the area or structure after locating it or performing the technique. Also respond to any questions that are posed. You will need a stethoscope.

Thorax

☐ Palpate the sternum and label Fig. 11–1.

   ☐ Palpate the sternoclavicular joint to rule out pathology of this structure.

   ☐ What three structures make up the sternum?

☐ Locate the ribs.

   ☐ Palpate each accessible rib and its costal cartilage. Remember that ribs 11 and 12 do not have anterior attachment via the costal cartilage.

   ☐ Which ribs are protected posteriorly by the scapula?

Abdomen

☐ Auscultate the abdomen.

   ☐ Place the stethoscope over the four abdominal quadrants (Fig. 11–2), and listen for the normal gurgling noises produced by peristalsis in a healthy digestive system.

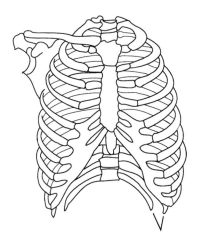

Figure 11–1 The thorax. (From Starkey, C, and Ryan, J: Evaluation of Orthopedic and Athletic Injuries, ed 2. FA Davis, Philadelphia, 2002, p 395, with permission.)

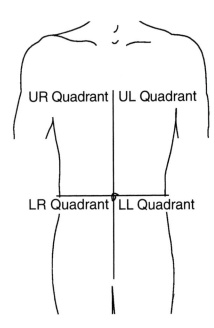

Figure 11–2 Abdominal quadrant reference system. (From Starkey, C, and Ryan, J: Evaluation of Orthopedic and Athletic Injuries, ed 2. FA Davis, Philadelphia, 2002, p 400, with permission.)

☐ Palpate the abdomen.

    ☐ With your partner in the hook-lying position, palpate each quadrant. The noninjured abdomen is pliable and not painful with palpation.

    ☐ What commonly injured structures are located in each of the following quadrants?

        ☐ Upper right quadrant _____

        ☐ Upper left quadrant _____

        ☐ Lower right quadrant _____

        ☐ Lower left quadrant _____

☐ Percuss the abdomen.

    ☐ Place your hand palm down over the structure to be assessed.

    ☐ Use the index and middle fingers of your other hand to tap the distal interphalangeal (DIP) joints of the hand already on your partner.

    ☐ Note the hollow resonant sound when percussing over most of the noninjured abdomen. Keep in mind that percussing over a solid organ (e.g., the liver) or over an area of internal bleeding will elicit a dull thump instead.

ACTIVITY 3   Thorax and Abdomen: Vital Sign Assessment

Instructions ➤ This exercise is designed to improve your vital sign assessment skills. Vital signs are included here because injury to this area may cause hemorrhage of vital organs that will adversely affect vital signs. Complete the following, placing a check next to the area as you complete it. Respond to any questions posed. You will need a stethoscope and sphygmomanometer.

Heart Rate

☐ Locate the pulse of the carotid artery just lateral to the thyroid cartilage.
☐ Count the number of pulsations occurring in 15 seconds.
☐ Multiply this number times 4 to obtain the beats per minute (bpm).
☐ Reassess the heart rate after your partner has exercised (e.g., running in place, jumping jacks) for 1 minute. Note the change in frequency and intensity of the pulse.
☐ What is a normal range for an athlete's resting heart rate?

Respiratory Rate

☐ Assess your partner's rate of breathing at rest.
☐ Then assess your partner's respiratory rate after a 1-minute bout of exercise.
☐ What is a normal respiratory rate?

Blood Pressure

☐ With your partner sitting or lying supine, secure the blood pressure cuff (sphygmomanometer) over the upper arm. Align any arrow on the cuff with the brachial artery. Be sure the arm is relaxed.
☐ Place the diaphragm of the stethoscope over the brachial artery.
☐ Inflate the cuff to 180 to 200 mm Hg.
☐ Slowly release the air from the cuff.
☐ Watch the gauge while you listen through the stethoscope. Note the number at which the first pulse sound is heard. This is the systolic pressure.
☐ Continue to slowly release the air, and note the value at which the last pulse is heard. This is the diastolic pressure.
☐ Reassess the blood pressure after your partner exercises for 1 minute. What changes did you find?
☐ What are the upper systolic and diastolic limits of normal blood pressure?

ACTIVITY 4   Skill Integration: Thorax and Abdomen

Scenario A male ice hockey player comes to the athletic training room complaining of abdominal pain of 2 days' duration. Explain and demonstrate your evaluation of this athlete. The model will not respond to your questions but will perform any actions that you request.

Optional: You have _____ minutes to complete your evaluation.

Evaluation

Name: _____ *Date:* _____

History		
Establishes mechanism of injury	YES ☐	NO ☐
Establishes date/time of injury	YES ☐	NO ☐
Establishes prior history (e.g., abdominal surgery)	YES ☐	NO ☐
Establishes location/type of pain (including any referred pain)	YES ☐	NO ☐
Questions for presence of the following:		
Nausea/vomiting	YES ☐	NO ☐
Blood in urine	YES ☐	NO ☐
Painful urination	YES ☐	NO ☐
Referred pain ("Pain anywhere else?")	YES ☐	NO ☐
Normal bowel movement	YES ☐	NO ☐
Establishes eating/drinking pattern since onset of symptoms	YES ☐	NO ☐
Establishes most comfortable position	YES ☐	NO ☐
Establishes presence/absence of painful breathing	YES ☐	NO ☐

Inspection		
Exposes area	YES ☐	NO ☐
Inspects for the following:		
Discoloration	YES ☐	NO ☐
Swelling	YES ☐	NO ☐
General posture	YES ☐	NO ☐
Auscultates abdomen	YES ☐	NO ☐

Palpation		
Has athlete assume supine, hook-lying position	YES ☐	NO ☐
Palpates for presence of the following:		
Pain	YES ☐	NO ☐
Rigidity/muscle guarding	YES ☐	NO ☐
Rebound tenderness	YES ☐	NO ☐
Palpates all four quadrants	YES ☐	NO ☐
Percusses abdomen	YES ☐	NO ☐

Functional Tests		

Student should note that results of these tests will be appropriately documented. Response is not correct if assessment is performed incorrectly. Examiner may wish to check the model's blood pressure before the student begins the assessment.

Vital signs assessment:

Blood pressure	YES ☐	NO ☐
Pulse rate	YES ☐	NO ☐
Respiratory rate	YES ☐	NO ☐

Presentation

Performs evaluation in a confident, professional manner ....YES ☐   NO ☐

Performs evaluation in a logical sequence ....YES ☐   NO ☐

Performs evaluation within allotted time ....YES ☐   NO ☐

TOTAL: _____ / _____

Evaluator: _____

Comments: _____

_____

_____

ACTIVITY 5   Eye: History

Instructions ➤   Have your partner select a common acute injury or condition of the eye. Ask a series of questions in an attempt to narrow the injury possibilities and guide the assessment. Your partner should provide the answers that would be likely from an athlete who sustained this injury or condition. Record all questions and responses, and discuss your conclusions with your partner and instructor. Repeat the process using a chronic injury.

Acute Injury

Question: _____

Response: _____

Question: _____

Response: _____

Question: _____

Response: _____

Question: _____

Response: _____

Question: _____

Response: _____

Question: _____

Response: _____

Question: _____

Response: _____

Question: _____

Response: _____

Question: _____

Response: _____

Question: _____

Response: _____

Chronic Injury

Question: _____

Response: _____

Question: _____

Response: _____

Question: _____

Response: _____

Question: _____

Response: _____

Question: _____

Response: _____

Question: _____

Response: _____

Question: _____

Response: _____

Question: _____

Response: _____

Question: _____

Response: _____

Question: _____

Response: _____

ACTIVITY 6   Eye: Inspection

Instructions ➤   Define the deformities, abnormalities, and conditions listed here. Inspect your partner's face and related structures to identify each condition. Because most of these conditions will not be found in the uninjured class population, find a photograph of the deformity in your textbook.

Foreign bodies _____

Orbital hematoma (black eye) _____

Enophthalmos (posterior displaced globe) _____

Exophthalmus (anteriorly displaced globe) _____

Stye _____

Hyphema _____

Subconjunctival hematoma _____

Conjunctivitis (pink eye) _____

Anisocoria _____

Unequal size   _____

Unequal shape   _____

Elliptical or teardrop   _____

ACTIVITY 7   Eye: Special Tests

Instructions ➤   This exercise is designed to improve skills involved in evaluating the injured eye. Complete the following using your partner as a model, placing a check next to the area after completing the technique. Respond to any of the questions posed. You will need an eye chart, a fluorescein strip, sterile saline, a cobalt-blue light, an ophthalmoscope, and a penlight if available.

☐ Palpate the infraorbital rim.
    ☐ Damage to what nerve can result in numbness in the cheek and lateral nose?

☐ Assess vision.
    ☐ Using a Snellen chart, determine your partner's visual acuity, with and without any corrective lenses.

☐ Assess pupil reaction to light.
    ☐ Have your partner hold his or her hand in front of the eye not being tested.
    ☐ Shine a penlight into the test eye for 1 second.
    ☐ Observe for pupil constriction and subsequent dilation once the light source is removed. Remember that some people have pupils that are naturally unequal sizes (anisocoria).

☐ Test with a fluorescein strip.
    ☐ Moisten strip with sterile saline.
    ☐ Touch the strip to the lower eyelid, being careful to avoid the cornea.
    ☐ Use the blue light to observe for any blue-green stain, indicative of a corneal or scleral abrasion. (Unless your partner has been injured, you probably will not see anything.)

☐ Observe eye motility.
    ☐ Look for symmetry of motion as your partner's eyes sweep through their range of motion.

☐ Remove contact lenses.
    ☐ Practice removing lenses on your classmates who wear them.
    ☐ Remove hard lens:
        ☐ Have partner open eyes as wide as possible.
        ☐ Pull outer margin of eyelid laterally.
        ☐ Hold your hand under the eye to catch the lens, and ask your model to blink. This should force the lens out of the eye.
    ☐ Remove soft lenses:
        ☐ Ask your partner to look upward. (Lifts part of lens off cornea.)
        ☐ Place your finger on the raised portion of the contact lens.
        ☐ Manipulate the lens inferiorly and laterally to a position where you can pinch it and safely remove it from the eye.

ACTIVITY 8   Face and Related Structures: History

Instructions ➤ Have your partner select a common acute injury involving the face or related structures. Ask a series of questions in an attempt to narrow the injury possibilities and guide the assessment. Your partner should provide the answers that would be likely from an athlete who sustained this injury. Record all questions and responses, and discuss your conclusions with your partner and instructor. Repeat the process using a chronic injury.

Acute Injury

Question: _____

Response: _____

Question: _____

Response: _____

Question: _____

Response: _____

Question: _____

Response: _____

Question: _____

Response: _____

Question: _____

Response: _____

Question: _____

Response: _____

Question: _____

Response: _____

Question: _____

Response: _____

Question: _____

Response: _____

Chronic Injury

Question: _____

Response: _____

Question: _____

Response: _____

Question: _____

Response: _____

Question: _____

Response: _____

Question: _____

Response: _____

Question: _____

Response: _____

Question: _____

Response: _____

Question: _____

Response: _____

Question: _____

Response: _____

Question: _____

Response: _____

ACTIVITY 9   Face and Related Structures: Inspection

Instructions ➤ Define the deformities, abnormalities, and conditions listed here. Inspect your partner's face and related structures to identify each condition. Because most of these conditions will not be found in the uninjured class population, find a photograph of the deformity in your textbook.

Ear

Auricular hematoma (cauliflower ear) _____

Battle's sign _____

Nose

Epistaxis _____

Raccoon eyes _____

Saddle nose deformity _____

Face and Jaw

Ecchymosis (black eye) _____

Bell's palsy _____

Malocclusion of teeth _____

Instructions ➤ Write the letter of the term in the left-hand column next to the corresponding description or injury implication in the right-hand column. Use each letter only once.

_____ 1. Auricular hematoma   A. Black eye

_____ 2. Battle's sign   B. Necrosis of nasal cartilage

_____ 3. Epistaxis   C. Cauliflower ear

_____ 4. Raccoon eyes   D. Nose bleed

_____ 5. Saddle nose deformity   E. Nasal fracture

_____ 6. Infraorbital ecchymosis   F. Nerve damage

_____ 7. Bell's palsy   G. TMJ dislocation

_____ 8. Malocclusion of teeth   H. Skull fracture

Instructions ➤ Inspect the ear and nose with the aid of an otoscope. Place a check next to the area after noting the structures or injury conditions listed here.

Ear (Attach Speculum)

☐ Cerumen
☐ Tympanic membrane

Nose

☐ Deviated septum

ACTIVITY 10   Face and Related Structures: Palpation

Instructions ➤ Review the discussion of bony anatomy (Fig. 11–3) and the sections on palpation in your textbook before completing this exercise. Begin by locating each landmark listed here on a skeleton, using the help of your textbook when needed. Develop a systematic approach so that no important structures are missed. Complete the remainder of the assignment after taking a break.

Without the aid of your textbook or skeleton, locate each landmark on your partner. When you have found the landmark, mark its location with a small sticker and place a check next to the landmark listed here. Use available resources (e.g., textbook, skeleton, instructor) to check the accuracy of your palpation.

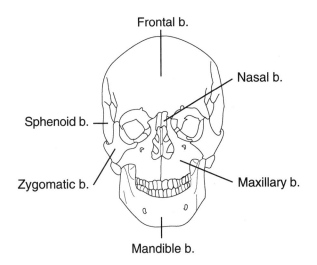

Figure 11–3 Bony anatomy of the face. (From Starkey, C, and Ryan, J: Evaluation of Orthopedic and Athletic Injuries, ed 2. FA Davis, Philadelphia, 2002, p 584, with permission.)

☐ Nasal bone
☐ Nasal cartilage
☐ Zygoma
☐ Maxilla
☐ Temporomandibular joint
☐ Periauricular area
☐ External ear
☐ Teeth
☐ Mandible
☐ Hyoid bone
☐ Cartilages (tracheal, cricoid, and thyroid)

ACTIVITY 11   Face and Related Structures: Special Tests

Introduction

Certain specific injuries and conditions, such as otitis media, require special tests that do not fit into the other assessment categories. These are often designed to stress a specific structure through scripted movements.

Instructions ➤ Provide the name for or describe (if there is no specific name) the special test or tests that may be used to identify the injuries and conditions listed here. Complete the special tests using your partner as the injured athlete. Describe a positive sign, and record this information in the space provided. If more than one blank is included, provide alternative tests.

Injury/Condition	Special Test	Positive Sign
Otitis media	_____	_____
Mandibular fracture	_____	_____
TMJ dislocation	_____	_____

ACTIVITY 12   Environmental Conditions: History

Instructions ➤ Have your partner select a heat-related condition that was discussed in your textbook. Ask a series of questions in an attempt to identify susceptibility to heat illness, narrow the condition possibilities, and guide the assessment. Your partner should provide the answers that would be likely from an athlete who sustained this condition. Record all questions and responses, and discuss your conclusions with your partner and instructor.

Question: _____

Response: _____

Question: _____

Response: _____

Question: _____

Response: _____

Question: _____

Response: _____

Question: _____

Response: _____

Question: _____

Response: _____

Question: _____

Response: _____

Question: _____

Response: _____

Question: _____

Response: _____

Question: _____

Response: _____

ACTIVITY 13   Environmental Conditions: Inspection and Palpation

Instructions ➤ Visually inspect and, if needed, manually palpate for each of the signs listed here. Check the boxes when you have correctly identified the implication of the signs.

	Signs	Implication
Skin	☐ Cool, moist, and pale	_____
	☐ Hot, dry, and red	_____
	☐ Cold, waxy, and red	_____
	☐ Cold, waxy, and pale	_____
Muscle tone	☐ Cramps	_____
	☐ Shivering	_____
	☐ Motor impairment	_____
	☐ Extreme motor impairment	_____
Pupils	☐ Dilated	_____
	☐ Decreased responsiveness to light	_____

ACTIVITY 14   Environmental Conditions: Sling Psychrometer

Instructions ➤ Use the sling psychrometer to determine temperature and relative humidity. Compare your results with reports from local weather services. Apply these results to the following chart to determine whether conditions are safe for play.

Dry Bulb Temperature, °F	Wet Bulb Temperature, °F	Humidity, %	Consequences
80 to 90	68	<70	No extraordinary precautions are required for athletes not predisposed to heat injury. Athletes who are predisposed (e.g., unconditioned, unacclimated, or losing more than 3% of body weight from water loss) require close observation.
80 to 90	69 to 79	>70	Regular rest breaks are necessary.
90 to 100		<70	Loose, breathable clothing should be worn, and wet uniforms require regular changing.
90 to 100	>80	>70	Practice should be shortened and modified. The use of protective equipment covering the body should be curtailed.
>100	>82		Practice should be canceled.

Guidelines for modification of athletic competition in hot or humid environments. (From Starkey, C, and Ryan, J: Evaluation of Orthopedic and Athletic Injuries, ed 2. FA Davis, Philadelphia, 2002, p 660, with permission.)

ACTIVITY 15   Cardiopulmonary Conditions: History

Instructions ➤ Have your partner select a cardiopulmonary condition that was included in your textbook. Ask a series of questions in an attempt to narrow the cardiopulmonary condition possibilities and guide the assessment. Your partner should provide the answers that would be likely from an athlete who has this condition. Record all questions and responses, and discuss your conclusions with your partner and instructor.

Question: _____

Response: _____

Question: _____

Response: _____

Question: _____

Response: _____

Question: _____

Response: _____

Question: _____

Response: _____

Question: _____

Response: _____

Question: _____

Response: _____

Question: _____

Response: _____

Question: _____

Response: _____

Question: _____

Response: _____

ACTIVITY 16   Cardiopulmonary Conditions: Inspection and Palpation

Instructions ➤   Perform this activity under two conditions: with an unconscious patient and with a conscious patient. Visually inspect and, if needed, manually palpate to determine the ABCs in an unconscious athlete. Next, consider a conscious athlete and inspect and palpate for each of the signs listed here. Place a check in the boxes where included to indicate the presence of the sign, and describe the sign if you included it.

Unconscious Athlete

Airway	☐ Yes	☐ No
Breathing	☐ Yes	☐ No
	☐ Bradypnea	
	☐ Tachypnea	
Circulations	☐ Yes	☐ No
	☐ Bradycardia	
	☐ Tachycardia	

Conscious Athlete

Position of the athlete	☐ Clutching chest in pain	
	☐ Bent over with hands on knee to aid breathing	
	☐ Hands in closed chain position to aid breathing	
	☐ Sitting with elbows on knees and head hanging to aid breathing	
Skin color	☐ Pale or ashen	☐ Cyanosis
Airway	☐ Yes	☐ No
Breathing	☐ Yes	☐ No
	☐ Bradypnea	
	☐ Tachypnea	
Circulations	☐ Yes	☐ No
	☐ Bradycardia	
	☐ Tachycardia	
Sweating	☐ Profuse	
Responsive	☐ Yes	☐ No

ACTIVITY 17   Skill Integration: Cardiopulmonary Conditions

Scenario   A volleyball player collapses on the court midway through a game. You immediately approach her and determine that she is unconscious.

Evaluation

In detail, describe your actions.

_____

_____

_____

_____

_____

_____

_____

Activity 18   Practical Questions

Instructions ➤   After reading chapters in your textbook and completing the corresponding activities, complete the following questions using your lab partner as the patient. The performance evaluation sheets that follow can be used by your instructor to grade the quality of your response to each question.

1. Your patient has received a blow to the abdominal region and complains of generalized pain. Define the boundaries of the four abdominal quadrants on your patient, and palpate the abdomen. As you palpate, identify the major organs in the abdominal region that are commonly injured during athletic activities. Also identify any helpful landmarks or areas of referred pain for the organs identified.

2. Assess the vitals signs (heart rate, blood pressure, and respirations) for your subject in question 1. Provide the following in your answer: normal value ranges, name of equipment used, and an explanation of your actions.

3. Using only a penlight, assess the eye for pupil size and shape, motility, and pupillary reaction to light. Indicate what is a normal sign and what would be considered abnormal. Also provide the implications for abnormal signs.

4. Perform and describe special tests used to identify (1) otitis media and (2) mandibular fracture. Include the name for each test and what is a positive sign.

5. Name and palpate the bones and significant bony landmarks that make up the face and related structures.

6. Imagine your subject is divided into two equal halves. The right side of the body is suffering heat exhaustion, and the left side is suffering heat stroke. Inspect your patient, and provide the signs that would indicate the given condition.

7. Imagine that your patient is suffering hypothermia. Provide the indications of hypothermia for each of the following signs: pupils, pulse, blood pressure, respiration, muscular function, and mental status. If the signs differ based on the severity of hypothermia, include these differing signs.

8. To ensure that you are always prepared to manage life-threatening conditions, it will be necessary that your instructor conduct this activity without warning or

preparation. A CPR mannequin will be used as your patient. Assess airway, breathing, and circulation in an unconscious patient. Assume your patient is not breathing and there is no circulation. Perform CPR for 5 minutes.

PERFORMANCE EVALUATION SHEETS

1. *Your patient has received a blow to the abdominal region and complains of generalized pain. Define the boundaries of the four abdominal quadrants on your patient, and palpate the abdomen. As you palpate, identify the major organs in the abdominal region that are commonly injured during athletic activities. Also identify any helpful landmarks or areas of referred pain for the organs identified.*

   Performance evaluation

   Define boundaries of four quadrants _____

RUQ	**LUQ**
Right kidney _____	Left kidney _____
Liver _____	Spleen _____
Gallbladder _____	

RLQ	**LLQ**
Appendix _____	Colon _____
Colon _____	

Midline Area
Bladder _____

2. *Assess the vitals signs (heart rate, blood pressure, and respirations) for your subject in question 1. Provide the following in your answer: normal value ranges, name of equipment used, and an explanation of your actions.*

   Performance evaluation

   HEART RATE

Palpate carotid artery	_____
Count beats for 15 seconds	_____
Multiply by 4 to get beats/min	_____
Normal value range	_____

   BLOOD PRESSURE

   Proper terminology for the following:

Stethoscope	_____
Sphygmomanometer	_____
Patient positioning	_____
Cuff placement	_____
Placement of stethoscope over brachial artery	_____

Inflate cuff to 180 to 200 mm Hg	_____
Noted first sound as systolic	_____
Systolic pressure	_____
Noted last sound as diastolic	_____
Diastolic pressure	_____
Normal value ranges	_____

RESPIRATIONS

| Number of breaths/min | _____ |
| Normal value ranges | _____ |

3. *Using only a penlight, assess the eye for pupil size and shape, motility, and pupillary reaction to light. Indicate what is a normal sign and what would be considered abnormal. Also provide the implications for abnormal signs.*

Performance evaluation

SIZE AND SHAPE

_____ Used penlight to observe shape and size of pupils

_____ Normal sign: pupils equal in size and shape

_____ Abnormal signs

    _____ Unequal size or shape   _____ Implication: Brain injury
                                                  Congenital

    _____ Elliptical shape   _____ Implication: Corneal laceration
                                                  Ruptured globe

MOTILITY

_____ Asked athlete to follow tip of penlight through eye's ROM

_____ Normal sign: smoothly tracks penlight through full ROM

_____ Abnormal sign: nystagmus   Implication: Brain injury

PUPILLARY REACTION TO LIGHT

_____ Covered eye, then shined 'penlight on pupil

_____ Normal sign: constricts with light

_____ Abnormal sign: remains dilated   Implication: Brain injury

(Continued)

4. *Perform and describe special tests used to identify (1) otitis media and (2) mandibular fracture. Include the name for each test and what is a positive sign.*

Performance evaluation

	Description	Test	Positive Sign
Otitis media	_____	_____	_____
Mandibular fracture	_____	_____	_____
TMJ dislocation	_____	_____	_____

5. *Name and palpate the bones and significant bony landmarks that make up the face and related structures.*

Performance evaluation

	Name	Palpation
Nasal bone	_____	_____
Nasal cartilage	_____	_____
Zygoma	_____	_____
Maxilla	_____	_____
Temporomandibular joint	_____	_____
Periauricular area	_____	_____
External ear	_____	_____
Teeth	_____	_____
Mandible	_____	_____
Hyoid bone	_____	_____

6. *Imagine your subject is divided into two equal halves. The right side of the body is suffering heat exhaustion, and the left side is suffering heat stroke. Inspect your patient, and provide the signs that would indicate the given condition.*

Performance evaluation

Sign	Heat Exhaustion	Heat Stroke
Consciousness	_____ Conscious	_____ Unconscious
Sweating	_____ Profuse	_____ None
Skin temperature	_____ Cool	_____ Hot
Skin color	_____ Pale	_____ Red
Skin moisture	_____ Clammy	_____ Dry
Body temperature	_____ Normal	_____ Significantly increased
Pulse rate	_____ Rapid	_____ Rapid
Pulse strength	_____ Weak	_____ Strong

7. *Imagine that your patient is suffering hypothermia. Provide the indications of hypothermia for each of the following signs: pupils, pulse, blood pressure, respiration, muscular function, and mental status. If the signs differ based on the severity of hypothermia, include these differing signs.*

Performance evaluation

Pupils _____

Pulse _____

Blood pressure _____

Respiration _____

Muscular _____

_____

Mental status _____

_____

8. *To ensure that you are always prepared to manage life-threatening conditions, it will be necessary that your instructor conduct this activity without warning or preparation. A CPR mannequin will be used as your patient. Assess airway, breathing, and circulation in an unconscious patient. Assume your patient is not breathing and there is no circulation. Perform CPR for 5 minutes.*

Performance evaluation

ASSESSMENT

Airway _____

Breathing _____

Circulation _____

CPR

Rescue breaths:

  Depth _____

  Frequency _____

  Number _____

Cardiac compressions:

  Location _____

  Force _____

  Frequency _____

  Number _____

Reassessment of ABCs _____

ANSWER KEY

Activity 2

Abdomen

Right upper quadrant	Right kidney
	Liver
	Gallbladder
Left upper quadrant	Left kidney
	Spleen
Right lower quadrant	Appendix
	Colon
Left lower quadrant	Colon

Activity 3

Resting heart rate:	60 to 100 beats/min
Resting respiratory rate:	12 to 20 breaths/min
Blood pressure	
Systolic:	100 to 140 mm Hg
Diastolic:	65 to 90 mm Hg

Note: Well-conditioned athletes will have values near the low end of each range.

Activity 11

Injury/Condition	Special Test	Positive Sign
Otitis media	Weber test	Hear vibrations louder in affected ear
Mandibular fracture	Tongue blade test	Athlete unable to maintain firm bite or pain is elicited (or both)
TMJ dislocation	Athlete attempts to open and close mouth	Malocclusion of teeth or inability to open and close mouth

Activity 13

	Signs	Implication
Skin	☐ Cool, moist, and pale	Heat exhaustion
	☐ Hot, dry, and red	Heat stroke
	☐ Cold, waxy, and red	Mild hypothermia
	☐ Cold, waxy, and pale	Severe hypothermia
Muscle tone	☐ Cramps	Heat cramps
	☐ Shivering	Slight hypothermia
	☐ Motor impairment	Mild hypothermia
	☐ Extreme motor impairment	Severe hypothermia
Pupils	☐ Dilated	Severe hypothermia
		Heat stroke
	☐ Decreased responsiveness to light	Heat or cold injury